Kata Bunkai are like ghosts,
Everyone talks about, but few have seen.

SHIHAN-TE

The Bunkai
of Karate
Kata

YMAA Publication Center
Boston, Mass. USA

YMAA Publication Center
Main Office
4354 Washington Street
Boston, Massachusetts, 02131
1-800-669-8892 • www.ymaa.com • ymaa@aol.com

10 9 8 7 6 5 4 3 2 1

Drawings: Hans Decoz
Cover Design: Frank J. Segovia

Publisher's Cataloging in Publication
(Prepared by Quality Books Inc.)

Craig, John, 1938-
 Shihan-te : the bunkai of kata / by Darrell Craig and
Paul Anderson. — 1st ed.
  p. cm.
  Includes index.
  LCCN: 2002101835
  ISBN: 1-886969-84-4

 1. Karate.   2. Self-defense.   I. Anderson, Paul V.
II. Title.

GV1114.3.C73 2002   613.6'6
                           QBI02-200220

Disclaimer: The author and publisher of this material are NOT RESPONSI-
BLE in any manner whatsoever for any injury which may occur through reading
or following the instructions in this manual.

The activities, physical or otherwise, described in this material may be too
strenuous or dangerous for some people, and the reader(s) should consult a physi-
cian before engaging in them.

Printed in Canada

Contents

Dedication vii
Foreword ix
Acknowledgements xi
Chapter One: The Bunkai of Kata 1
    Why Write About Bunkai of Kata
    To Disassemble Kata
    Historical Context of Karate
    Kata Today in the Twenty-First Century
    The Triangle of Teaching
Chapter Two: Traditional Kata: The Lost Soul 25
    The Source of Kata
    The Secrecy Demanded of Kata
    The Oral Tradition of Karate Kata
    The Two Schools of Karate: Exhibition and Traditional
Chapter Three: Some Know Better 35
    Everything in Life is Kata
    The Modern Teaching of Old Ways
    Boxers and Ballerinas
    The Creeping Effect of Novice Teachers
    Kata's Staying Power
    Language, Translation, Misinterpretation and Ignorance
    Bunkai, Oyo, Henka and Kakushi
    Zanshin, Finishing With Attention
    See the Light or Feel the Heat
Chapter Four: The Four Elements of Kata: Bunkai, Oyo,
    Henka, Kakushi 51
    Bunkai, the First Element
    Oyo, the Second Element
    Henka, the Third Element
    Kakushi, the Fourth Element
    Capturing the Intended Sense
Chapter Five: Demonstrating the Four Elements of a Kata 59
    Demonstrating Bunkai
    Demonstrating Oyo
    Demonstrating Henka
    Demonstrating Kakushi
    Conclusion: The Practical Application of Bunkai
Chapter Six: Waza Descriptions 95
Chapter Seven: My Introduction to Kata 159
Glossary 163
Index 166

Dedication

This book is dedicated to all of the martial artists who have known the four weaknesses in their art:

Surprise, Fear, Confusion and Doubt.

The mind of a martial artist that takes a negative path, in kata, creates indecision, surprise and doubt. One leads progressively to the other in the untrained mind. It is our hope that this book, in some small way, will help bring union to your mind. Always remember that SOUND is first (then sight, and lastly feel). Lying between sound and sight is the bunkai, or technique. If you only have feel, your karate is not complete.

Foreword

More than two decades ago, during my first formal practice in karate, I was introduced to the practice of kata. It was very puzzling to me what good this 'little dance' was. Like many children attracted to the martial arts, I was dazzled by the flashy moves I had seen in the movies and the fearlessly calm power the martial arts hero seemed to have over his opponents. I had only a rudimentary understanding of meditation and visualization so I ascribed kata to these rarified realms of knowledge and trusted my sensei to be my guide. I wanted the combat, the demanding drills, the flashy new maneuver. Today, I wonder how my sensei had the patience and dedication to make a martial artist out of such ignorant enthusiasm, but I believe it was his belief in the truth of kata and its tradition as a means of transmission of the original data from the progenitor to the student untold years after his passing.

Years later, as a physical education professional, I have been exposed to many approaches and styles of educational theory and application. Each had its pluses and minuses, but all differentiated themselves from the previous theory by stating how it was different or better because of an emphasis on this concept, style or theory. Intrinsically, this kind of thinking is prejudicial and flawed. Consequently, I think that it was not only wise but also purifying to be exposed to the bunkai of kata free from the prejudices of one style or another. The bunkai the authors illuminate, free from name, nationality and nomenclature, validates itself allowing us to hold a mirror up to our own styles of kata, no matter the origin, and see the truth hidden therein.

I do not pretend to understand all the beauty and truth inherent in kata, but I thank the authors for opening my eyes. I still have a lifetime of practice ahead of me to find it and so do you.

Lanny D. Morton,
Coach, English teacher, and martial artist
Humble High School
Humble, Texas

Acknowledgements

I have worked on several movies, including *We Come in Peace*, *Challenger* (for which I was the technical advisor for martial arts), *Rush* (with Sam Elliot who was a wonderful person to work with), *RoboCop II*, and *Sidekicks*. In one of these movies an actor, promoted as a martial artist, could not perform a karate kick to the head despite repeated attempts to do so. As a consequence, the construction crew had to build him a special platform to stand on (which, of course, the camera never showed) so it would look like he had delivered the head kick. So much for what you see on the screen.

In the last century, there have been many great teachers that have possessed the intimate knowledge of kata. Several are even alive today. One of the most influential knowledgeable senseis that I has come across in a long time is Yamazaki Sensei from the Ryobukai. Credit must be given for his unfathomable patience, profound understanding of kata, and its traditional, intended purpose. He is certainly very knowledgeable about teaching many of the bunkai, as well as the kakushi and henka.

In closing I want to recognize three people who were so instrumental in this undertaking. First, Ms. Claudia Smith without whose dedication, typing, input and above all, patience, this manuscript would only be half finished. Second, my co-author, Mr. Paul Anderson, whose research on the subject seemed to be unlimited. Lastly, Mr. Gary Grossman, who has been much more than a student but a close friend. He has brought life to these pages with his editing and understanding.

To all these people I say, "Thank You!"

Darrell Max Craig
Houston, Texas

Front of fan, "Gratitude and Principles,"
and signature of Ryoichi Sasagawa.

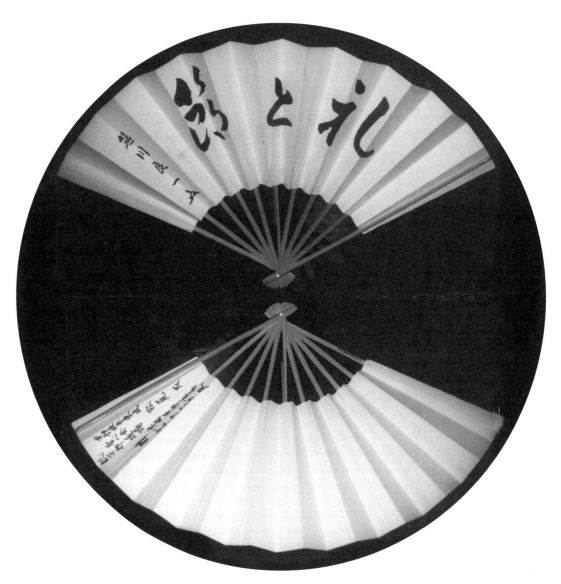

Back of fan:
"Presented to Darrell Craig
Beikoku-Honbu-Dojo
by Sigeru Matsuo
All Japan Karate Champion
Seison-Kai So Honbo Dojo

CHAPTER ONE

The Bunkai of Kata

WHY WRITE ABOUT BUNKAI OF KATA

There is irony in the writing of this book. First, it is about karate, which many years ago introduced me to the martial arts. Although karate was the art that opened the door for me to a whole world of wonderful people, a fascinating culture and a way of life, I have also written about three other arts before this: *iai*, which was the subject of *Iai, the Art of Drawing the Sword* (Charles E. Tuttle Company, Inc.), *jujitsu*, covered in *Japan's Ultimate Martial Art, Jujitsu Before 1882, The Classical Japanese Art of Self-Defense* (Charles F. Tuttle Company, Inc.) and *kendo*, which I covered in *The Heart of Kendo* (Shambhala Publications, Inc.).

Second, it is a book I said I would never write because there were already so many books on the subject. How, I wondered, is anyone going to differentiate this book from all the others on the shelves? I have read many of those books. A very few were quite good. The rest? Well, let's be charitable and say they had a point. But none, I noticed, ever touched on what I consider to be the heart of the art: traditional *kata* and, more specifically, the *bunkai* of kata. In my opinion, kata is the most vital element of karate, or of any martial art for that matter. It is kata that allows an art to be practiced effectively and handed down from generation to generation. Many books, of course, provided step-by-step instruction on how to complete a given sequence of movements. But none adequately explained the interrelationship between those moves and the hidden techniques for which they were designed. It is the purpose of this book to fill this critical void.

I do not know for sure, but I suspect that there are several reasons that no one has written adequately about karate kata and its bunkai. One reason was expressed to me years ago when I visited another sensei's dojo. "Do you do traditional kata here?" I asked. "Not in this dojo," was the reply. "Here we only spar; that's what karate is all about. Fighting. It's bad enough we have to learn some of it before testing. After that? Forget it." This sensei either did not appreciate the significance of traditional kata or had discarded it because his students did not want to do it—in effect, discarding a valued and essential ingredient for a lower goal: commercialism. Many students do not want to study kata because the limited amount of kata to which they are exposed in tournaments, they rightly label as showy and useless. They are correct about what they have seen in tournaments, however they are incorrect about traditional kata, which they seldom, if ever, see or experience. Nevertheless, because of the hidden nature of its *waza* techniques, they could not appreciate them anyway—not without some sort of formal training. Only with proper instruction will they be able to recognize what the untrained eye will not. Another reason why no one has written adequately on this topic is that, even in Japan, many of the old traditions have disappeared. As a consequence, there are many people writing about karate today who have never studied traditional kata and its bunkai. How could they be expected to write competently about something they literally know nothing about?

You'll notice that, throughout this preface, I have used the phrase "*traditional* kata." I emphasize the word "traditional," because virtually none of the kata you see in tournaments, dojos, and demonstrations today is what this book is about. So do not think that reading this book will help you win the blue ribbon. What you see in these competitions may be athletically impressive and flashy, with all sorts of spins, high kicks, splits and other maneuvers (it most assuredly is entertaining), but this is not true kata. Why? A seemingly frivolous but serious answer is that it was constructed from the wrong end. What you see in modern day kata was designed to emphasize the theatrical moves I mentioned.

Traditional kata started with, and was built around, the *hidden* moves—real time-tested techniques. These are known as the *bunkai*. These techniques had to be practiced, of course, in order for skills to be maintained and knowledge passed on. To do so, these bunkai were incorporated into a linked series of logically coherent moves that became the traditional kata. But first, each move or group of related moves were modified, sometimes slightly or sometimes grossly, so that the prying eyes of unintended observers could not discover the true lethal function. The end result was traditional kata.

Karate was introduced to Japan only in 1926, 15 years before the outbreak of the Second World War. During the war, the practice of karate in Japan declined substantially and, after the war, the practice of all martial arts was forbidden in Japan for a brief period. As a consequence, once the practice resumed, there was a shortage of qualified instructors. This gave rise to the "instant karate master." There are many stories of karate "instructors" who would take a lesson from a qualified instructor during the day and then, that same night, teach what they had just learned to a group of unsuspecting students. This phenomenon, which infected the Japanese arts in the 1950s, is now being repeated throughout the world. It is impossible to learn true, traditional karate from these ninety-day wonders. Learning true karate takes years of painstaking effort under the eyes and guidance of a true master. Only through such effort can one learn the katas of a particular style well enough so that the master will unlock and reveal the hidden secrets of the bunkai for the student.

Most of these self-appointed masters resort to some free form or otherwise simply fabricate "techniques" from the showy moves they may have read about or seen in movies or on television. Anyone who can move their limbs can duplicate these moves, but they have nothing to do with karate and are utterly useless from any perspective except as physical exercise. It never ceases to amaze me that people will accept as true what they see on television or in the movies. We hope this book will introduce a more realistic perspective.

One of the challenges with writing about any martial art is that the authors, more often than not, pigeonhole themselves to a specific brand or particular style and therefore, by default, exclude many more readers than a general subject article would. For example, the only people who subscribe to Corvette magazines are likely only those that own Corvettes. The authors of this book felt that by overtly and openly identifying the particular kata that they have written about, the reader would miss the point and their intentions. And so within the body of this book, we have chosen not to identify our style or any one style. Furthermore, we feel it is to the advantage of the reader not to even name the particular kata that we discuss in depth.

This book is not really intended for the beginner, but neither is it intended for the master of karate. It is our hope that this book will be helpful to those in karate who are still traveling the road to perfection. It is quite likely, however, that those *karateka* in the midst of their journey may have come across this particular kata at one time or another. For those readers, it must kept in mind that within their own style the definitions of the techniques, *bunkai*, *oyo*, *henka*, and *kakushi*, may not be exactly the same.

What is important is that the reader carefully studies the relationship between the kata as demonstrated and the underlying bunkai. Maybe, just maybe, if enough readers do so, we can begin to reverse the tragic misconceptions that exist with so many students today about—not only the exquisite beauty of kata—but also the critical importance of studying traditional kata in order to become a true karateka.

In the West, we are often motivated to study the art of karate as a means of individual self-expression. In Japan, however, traditional karate practitioners seek to eradicate their ego through their practice. To the vast majority of people who observe kata, this difference in purpose may seem imperceptible. To an expert, however, the same kata performed by practitioners with dissimilar attitudes will look strikingly different. I have always thought that cleaning the dojo floor, quietly doing makuso before and after practice, and the wearing of the white gi were all designed to create an environment in which one might better take control of one's ego. Keep in mind that the assertion of one's ego, or resistance to the discipline of karate, is usually the greatest obstacle in learning the art. If we look at ourselves truthfully, we find beings filled with jealously, anger, vanity and, we must not forget, pride. All of these feelings must be eliminated before you can truly say you practice traditional karate.

The old masters in their wisdom realized that the true mastery of their karate bunkai went hand in hand with the mastery of one's inner self. They knew that the discovery of the bunkai's secrets is only secondary to the self-mastery and perfection of one's own human character. And within the harsh discipline that old masters demanded, students unknowingly developed their inner selves as they practiced kata.

The ego is just an obstacle in the process of understanding the bunkai (self-defense) or truth in the kata. One must travel the endless road of karate to eliminate the ego, which in turn will allow one to extract the truth from the kata. Once one starts to extract the truth from each move in a particular kata, one will begin to acquire a state of mind called *mushin*, which means "no mind". Buddhists refer to this state as *satori*—one with enlightenment. When one reaches this state of mind, one will find a whole new world.

Opinions like those of senseis who believe that sparring is the only proper way to practice karate ring out consistently in dojos all over the world for novice karate students to overhear. Unfortunately, most of us in the martial arts have at one time or another harbored such misconceptions about kata. We believe that this is due primarily to two reasons. First, the students, and more times than not the teachers, have very little insight into kata's intent and purpose as well as its training application. This information is generally unavailable. In our search for such information through the karate books on the open market, we found little about the bunkai of kata and even when we did, the information was very vague and often even misleading. Secondly, it is a natural result of our lack of familiarity with the coherent yet complex system. This by itself cannot be condemned but when ignorance becomes the prevailing attitude, it becomes a malevolence that affects the growth of the art.

As we attended more and more karate tournaments and looked at the kata that was being performed, we felt something was wrong. The kata in most cases was meaningless, just a shadow of the past demonstrated in dance-like moves that were often dry and barren. Largely, kata have become nothing more than an exhibition. Most students have lost the bunkai or training application within the shadowy moves.

Confused about what exactly he was asked to judge at times, Craig Sensei came upon the idea of interviewing the oldest and most experienced sensei He could find on the subject. The opportunity, however, did not present itself until a visit with K. Fukuda, an 84-year old sensei who was not only eager to talk about the problem of modern day kata, but who was quite qualified to make the distinction as he had trained intensively under one of the founders of a particularly well-known system.

In that interview, the first thing that was pointed out to him was how far off the track modern kata had come in comparison to where it was when Fukuda Sensei first started training. Sensei pointed out numerous technical discrepancies in the modern kata. More than ever, he was convinced that the real bunkai in kata was not getting out to the modern karate student—not even from those senseis who themselves knew. Sensei came to the conclusion that the reason for this apparent laxness is not important. It is sufficient that the reader only realizes that the problem is real. Sensei Fukuda explained that all the great fighting systems of Okinawa and Japan were effective only because they were constructed from kata, whether they were systems of karate (empty hand) fighting or others. Under no circumstances were these great fighting arts developed by senseis who engaged just in mortal combat day after day. These old senseis constructed a normal process of walking before running in which the most effective movement and technique was first designed, then developed, tested, improved and finally standardized through the mode of artistic expression in kata. Kata should always precede sparring. In *kenjutsu*, it was always practiced intensively before the combat test of *shinken shobu* (dueling with real swords).

Each style of karate or martial arts system that expected to survive past its founder had to take the combinations of parts or elements from proven combative tests and used to build a cohesive system. This could only be done through kata, not through day-to-day combat. The student should always remember that the most essential part of kata is the technique or bunkai that is interwoven into the prearranged exercise. This means that the kata can teach the student the reasons why a technique will fail or succeed in *kumite* or, traditionally, in combat. It must always be kept in mind that in order to be able to find these hidden lessons within the katas, the karateka must evolve his kata out of the doing stage and into the using stage.

We feel the biggest misunderstanding about kata is a result of the fact that kata is a prearranged sequence of choreographed movements. To most students of martial arts and many inexperienced senseis, this prearranged exercise is practiced only to look good. Nothing could be further from the truth. With regard to this attitude, let us discuss the two developmental levels of kata: the doing and the using stages. Exhibition kata is largely a "doing" type kata while kata performed as a "using" type exercise will expose the effectiveness or shortcomings of techniques against an opponent. This is how it should be if kata is being practiced correctly. Kata is therefore an appraisal tool that allows the student to discover whether or not techniques are being applied correctly. More times than not, kata also reveals the reasons why the student or the techniques, or both, are failing to produce the desired result.

To Disassemble Kata

A kata can be taken apart like a piece of machinery. In fact, one of the translations of the word *bunkai* is "to disassemble." It is important to learn how each of part of a particular kata functions. This kind of analysis is known as bunkai, a much neglected form of study within karate. For the old masters, most of whom may have only practiced one or two kata their entire lives, the repetitions demanded of kata never became a burden because of the bunkai. As a student progresses from the introduction of a kata through a life of repetition, he will come to be exposed to the deeper and deeper inner and personal meanings behind the outward form.

When Fukuda Sensei was speaking of the prearranged disposition of kata, the subject came up about how many teachers and students wholly disregard kata in their training, believing that skills needed for sparring can be learned by kicking and punching a bag over and over until it becomes natural for defense or offense. Sensei then asked, "What would you call that type of workout or exercise?" I thought for a minute, and then said, "Well, I guess you call it *uchikomi*." "...Right! And uchikomis are nothing but prearranged kata. So there you are, those students are doing kata whether they realize it or not by repeating certain movements against their more or less cooperative self."

In this book, we wish to alert the reader to the fact that unless you know each and every bunkai (technique) for any particular kata movement, you cannot hope to ever perform the kata correctly. Only competent senseis who wish to teach the hidden bunkai in their kata can guide you in your quest for that perfection. Many karateka complain that much of a particular kata is subject to their sensei's interpretation. They become confused when one sensei says or demonstrates one thing and another says or demonstrates something else. This is a relevant situation so I will try to address it. Old traditional or at least technical kata in most karate *ryu*, also known as styles or schools, are standardized. There is a technically correct way of performing them, but you must also keep in mind that from decade to decade there is a natural, gradual process of change.

The All Japan and All Okinawan Karate Federations, in some cases, have changed some parts of the katas from their founders' time. There have been modifications to, and in some instances an actual changing of, the waza itself in order to be more adaptable to modern times. In most cases, the federations sought and attained the approval of the majority of karate masters before deviating from the original kata. Therefore karate senseis who are not up-to-date on this standardization may be using the older concept of the kata. Unfortunately, it is often the case that variations that do not make sense are the result of personalized variations and the lack of knowledge on the part of the teacher.

Here again I must stress how important it is to select a qualified sensei who is up to date on all the changes. Along these lines you must also keep in mind that traditional karate kata, while standardized, is not the only karate kata in existence. There are numerous high-ranking karate senseis that have established their own interpretations of a certain ryu's kata. I personally feel that it is not a matter of which katas are wrong or right, but understanding that this move can exist in different directions. The most important thing for the student to understand is that these standardized kata exist.

Kata is in my opinion the most vital ingredient of karate, or any martial art. It allows the art to mature, grow and develop as a system along with you as an individual. Kata must be emphasized, not as a demonstration but as a training method. The truth about karate kata is not being placed before the students of the world and I feel they have every right to label, most of the time, what they see at today's tournaments as something weak and almost useless. These same students are right about the de-emphasis being placed on kata today but they are not right about the true traditional kata. As someone once said, "It is a case of the singer, not the song."

HISTORICAL CONTEXT OF KARATE

Traditional karate is over one thousand years old. Think about that statement and ask yourself how an invisible edifice built by man, with no walls and no floor, can last a thousand years? Answer: kata and its hidden bunkai. At the same time keep in mind, sport karate has only been practiced for a few decades.

Many new students ask where karate came from and who started it all? Many people erroneously believe that karate is a traditional Japanese martial art. It is not. Traditional Japanese arts were the arts of the samurai. They were highly skilled in the use of their bodies as a weapon, but this was through the art of jujitsu. The samurai were well versed in precisely how to choke, or how to twist a joint which, when coupled with a waza, would produce a devastating effect. Interestingly, it was against the samurai code to use their fists in settling a dispute, believing that this type of brawling was fit for only the lower classes.

There are many stories about the origins of karate, but I feel it is most important for the reader to know that almost all Okinawan karate is credited to the Fukien Shaolin Temple in China. Chinese boxing was introduced to Okinawa as *Tode* (Chinese hand) and became labeled as *Shuri-Te*, *Tomari-Te* and *Naha-Te* then fragmented into the various modern-day styles of karate.

In 1922, two Okinawan karate masters by the names of Choki Motobu and Gichin Funikoshi went to Osaka and Tokyo in Japan to find out the Japanese judgment on the merits of Okinawan karate, which was then actually called *Okinawa Te*. It was, however, not until 1926 that Gichin Funikoshi returned with a few students and introduced his art to Japanese budo masters. This demonstration of karate was the introduction and the beginning of the spread of Okinawa Te throughout the world.

It is interesting to note that it was not until after the eighteenth century, because of its secrecy, that Okinawa Te had any clear classifications as to various styles and types. As well, before 1926, karate as we have come to know it was called simply *Te* or Hand. The Japanese in that era referred to it as Okinawa Te. The two ideograms that were used to describe Okinawa Te actually read Chinese Hand. Sometime after 1926 and when Okinawa Te was accepted and adopted into the Japanese budo system, the Japanese changed the ideograms from Chinese Hand to Kara (empty) Te (hand) by which the world has come to know it. In the West, we have the tendency to pronounce karate, *ka-rahtee*, which is incorrect. The proper way to pronounce karate is *kara-tay*.

Okinawa sits 750 miles from the mainland of Japan and though at one time it had its kings and queens, Okinawan warriors were never looked upon by the Japanese as the equals of Japanese samurai by any stretch of the imagination. The Okinawans were a conquered people and the Japanese samurai ruled. I think this misunderstanding comes from the word *bushi*. On the mainland of Japan a bushi means samurai, but in Okinawa it refers to someone who has mastered all the movements of a karate kata and discovered the correct path of karate. The same word and spelling, but with two completely different meanings in Japan and Okinawa.

The Okinawans were mostly fishermen and farmers with an influx of trade from China and the Philippines. This port of call was vital to Japan's intercourse with the rest of the world. The Japanese ruled with swords in the daytime, the Okinawans ruled with hands and feet by night. The Okinawans in today's society believe that the banning of weapons by one of their first kings was a sublime act of wisdom, not one of oppression. Through this ban of weapons, the Okinawans developed a culture within their family units and a fighting system for their own exclusive use. Family fighting systems were closely guarded from any outsider.

Out of these family systems of self-defense came the fighting philosophy of *issen-issatsu* or "one strike". The purpose was to defend against opponents who were more heavily armed than themselves as in the case of visiting Chinese or Philippine seamen. The development of the ability to take a life in one strike was indeed necessary. The physical ability to take a life in one strike is practiced in *waza* and *keiko*. However, the psychological ability is developed through kata training. These two techniques essentially define Okinawan karate. Night training and the accompanying secrecy of karate ended in 1875 or thereabouts with the withdrawal of the Satsuma Samurai that had ruled for over 300 years. Okinawa was officially recognized as a part of Japan. It is also interesting to note that it was not until around 1904 or 1905 that karate actually became popularly known through its introduction as a physical education requirement in the Okinawan public schools. The old Okinawan karate masters believed that their kata could instill the proper discipline and character their children needed. The competitive aspects of karate were thought at that time to be unessential and unnecessary.

Looking back at the history of karate, kendo, and judo, we think it is ironic in our modern society that it is the competitive aspects of these arts that have kept them alive and thriving for such a long time. Even though karate was taught in the public schools, it was still an art past down from generation to generation through hand to hand teaching combined with oral tradition. Even with the written evidence that Okinawa is over 1000 years old, it is hard to find any written material on the history of karate. This may have come about because of World War II, but I feel that with the ban of weapons for the second time by the Japanese Satsuma clan in 1609, the art of karate went deep underground and was handed down from father to son in utmost secrecy. Therefore, very little was put down on paper.

KATA TODAY IN THE TWENTY-FIRST CENTURY

As we arrive in the twenty-first century, we feel that the desire to excel in the martial arts for self-defense and self-discipline still exists. A person strives initially today in the martial arts to become a black belt. The student should keep in mind as their training progresses that they should become aware of a stronger calling; the molding of themselves into a better person with honor and dignity, not just the ability to win over one's opponent. We must always keep in mind that youth is like a butterfly's dream and only lasts a short time. Old age is with us a lifetime. When one becomes a black belt without knowing the depth of the kata's bunkai, he or she has nothing to give to the student who is searching for the truth. The black belt should be an award given to the modern samurai who has sacrificed numerous hours to the honing of his body and mind with the discipline that kata demands. The black belt is supposed to be a symbol of an expert who has achieved not only the physical and mental aspects of the art, but the secrets of its kata as well.

Kata is a combat with oneself. Every movement of its bunkai is adapted for a specific situation. Only those black belts who can identify their opponent's attack and fight against it, only those who can look into their opponent's every move and thought will be able to react appropriately. These black belts are true students of kata. The student who is searching for the true path of karate will find that every traditional kata begins with a defensive action. This by itself demonstrates the peaceful nature of the training. It is a training with no aggressive purpose; only one that is based on the students' total control of themselves.

In our years of studying karate, we have come to realize that there is a huge disparity between different systems in regard to the standards they expect a black belt to meet. Originally the ranking system was established for the sole purpose of providing a reference by which the sensei could distinguish between the advanced or beginner student. There was not a sequence of colored belts in the beginning. It was white until the sensei changed it to black. In Japan you were a *kyu*, low step, until you reached the *dan* grade, high step. This type of ranking system introduced by Dr.

Jigaro Kana, the founder of judo, has worked well in motivating the student, but unfortunately it has developed some problems.

One of the main problems within the karate ranking system stems mainly from the fact that there are so many different styles or schools, each having its own set of standards when it comes to testing. When karate spread throughout the world, each country that embraced a style established its own set of standards. This made possible a situation that exists throughout the world of karate today in which unscrupulous individuals have been able to set up their own organizations through which they hand out black belts to many unqualified students. These students in turn decide to set up their own schools and hand out their own black belts. These are the same people that also decide to promote themselves to higher ranks for financial gain. Most people who sign up their children with a karate school never ask questions like, "Where did you learn your art?" or "How long have you been in business?" or "Do you do this for a living or just part time?" Even if they did ask these questions, they most likely would not understand the answers. The public is unaware of the difference in ranking and ability of a true black belt. These parents are easily lured into schools which award rank by credit card or promise a black belt to the student in a short period of time, maybe even one or two years. This not only degrades the quality of karate, and is also very dangerous to the student who gains a false sense of security.

The prospective student should be wary of those schools that use the word "black belt" as a come-on to cheat and defraud people out of their money. It should take anywhere from three to five years of hard work to earn a black belt from a respectable school, and then only under a competent instructor. Receiving a *shodan* grade (first grade of black belt) in three years is like receiving a college associate's degree; in four years, like a bachelor's degree; in five years, like a masters degree, and so on. I feel it's important to educate the public about the significance of the black belt and make the prospective student understand that the black belt is not a gift but a goal, a symbol of one's great dedication and effort.

Kendo and judo have one international standard of testing which pretty much prevails throughout the world. Most likely this is due in part to the fact that both have their origins in Japan where the rules of rank grew with the art itself. Unfortunately, the black belt will not always represent an expert. The samurai of old allowed nothing to tarnish their honor. He knew that his sword was never sharpened but was polished to perfection to receive the perfect cutting edge. Should the karate senseis of today desire anything less?

THE TRIANGLE OF TEACHING

As we look back, there is one thing we are sure of: in the beginning, the true Way, or *dō,* of kata cannot be followed without a proper teacher. The teacher, however, cannot train you in the way. He can only show the way through his own examples and watch you as you find your own path. As Miyamoto Musashi once said, "The teacher is as a needle, the disciple is as thread." (Musashi, *A Book of Five Rings*, Translated by Victor Harris, Overlook Press 1974 p.41)

Who is more important, the teacher or the student? Kata requires three things: a teacher, a student and a will to learn. Senseis say that it takes three things to make a dojo: the teacher, the student and the teacher's teacher. *There is a triangle.* The teacher cannot teach without having somebody to teach him, the student cannot learn without the teacher, and eventually the student becomes a teacher. It is a powerful circle when held together.

In the beginning when one starts practicing the martial arts, the teacher is the most important element. He is the one that knows how and when to apply critical motivations—sparks to help keep a student going. Sparks are needed particularly at moments when you are asked to do boring, repetitious processes and techniques whose purpose is totally foreign to you. In fact, the hardest thing to do if you are a martial artists is to just come to the school at the time you are supposed to—one, two or three times a week for a couple of years. Good students must learn to endure on their sensei's encouragement alone. A little spark at that right moment to get you over a hump—that is the job of a good instructor.

However, teachers must be very careful that, as they feed their students, they do not feed them too much. Students must be kept lean, and their minds need to be fed just enough so that they can get over these inevitable humps. And a teacher must take care, because if he does not, he may only see masses of students coming in and out of his school like a river that just keeps refilling the dojo. A poor teacher falls into the trap of substituting activity for achievement. In proven, venerable and traditional schools, the students of today always include students from yesterday; students who started fifteen or twenty years ago.

Kata is a foreign concept to many people, but what it teaches you is endurance, stamina and the challenges of character. An excellent teacher guides you through what the martial arts is really about. Ironically, in time, the student becomes more important because then the teacher begins to rely on the student to provide spark and motivation. No matter what a teacher says or what you learn from a kata, the ultimate teacher is yourself. In time, the lessons to be learned from kata are taught by oneself.

In the beginning. the student trying to learn kata is desperate to follow the teacher's instructions. The student's mind is so clouded with simply trying to perform kata correctly, that he has absolutely no concept of what he is actually doing. At an advanced level, the student should not be doing anything. He should project himself into the kata as though into an empty cup; a cup that has already been filled and that he has already consumed. Then he can now just let the subconscious mind take a hold of the kata's intention and perform the kata to perfection.

Eventually, kata becomes subconscious. One of Darrell Craig's teachers would come to visit from Japan and stay at his home. In the morning, Mr. Craig would go to wake up his sensei and would find him sound asleep and snoring, but amazingly with his hands together, waving around in the air doing kata! When one does kata in one's sleep, when you breath it, you sleep it, and you really live it; this is when you are really a master.

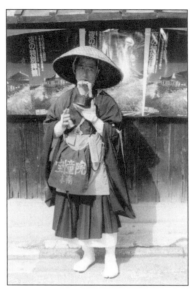

Trip to Japan in 1988 to O-sensei's
grave at Omura (Nagasaki).

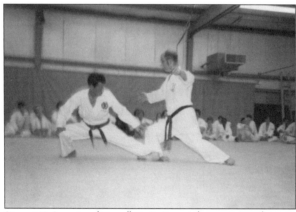

Siyogoi K. Sensei and Darrell Craig Sensei demonstrating the
bunkai to an advanced karate kata.

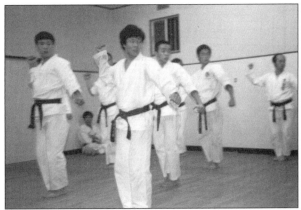

Osaka Hombu Dojo students performing Peian Godan kata.

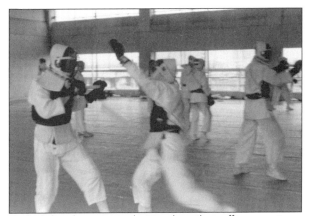

Osaka Police department taiho jitsu class. These officers practice three times a day for one hour, Monday through Friday. This photo was taken in the late 1970s when Darrell Craig was practicing advanced police training in Japan.

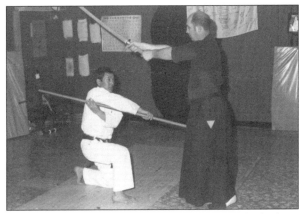

Siyogoi K. Sensei and Darrell Craig Sensei practicing the bunkai for a bo kata.

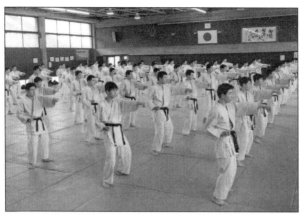

The Japanese Police Academy in Osaka, Japan. These officers are practicing a karate punching kata. Darrell Craig spent two days with Masao Fukuda Sensei, instructor with the Central Japan Police Schools.

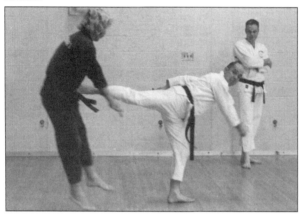

Darrell Craig at a karate tournament in the late 1970s.

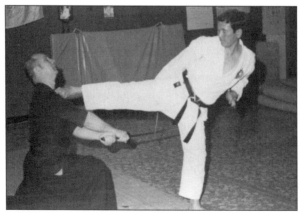

Siyogoi K. Sensei and Darrell Craig practicing the bunkai with the sai. If you look closely you will see that the sai are actually blocking the sword behind Sensei's thigh.

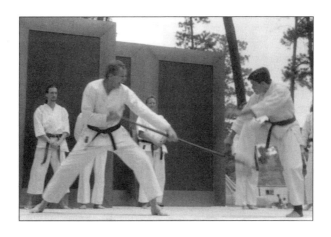

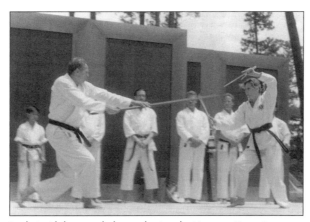

Bunkai with bo, nunchaku, and sai at the Houston, Texas Japanese Festival. The Budokan students performing are Tim Mousel with the bo, Ryan Clarke with nunchaku and Jeana Christ with the sai.

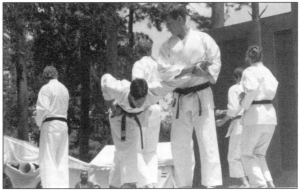

Mark Oberkirch and Ryan Clacke performing karate bunkai at the Houston Japanese Festival. We include this photograph because it demonstrates the same movement as in Figures 23 and 35.

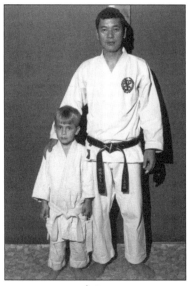

My son Darren with Siyogoi K. Sensei. Darren is now a nidan in judo and a sandan in kendo.

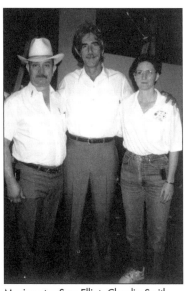

Movie actor Sam Elliot, Claudia Smith, and myself on the set of the movie Rush.

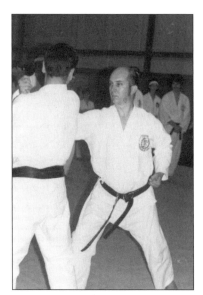

K. Siyogo Sensei demonstrating a waza from a kata with Darrell Craig.

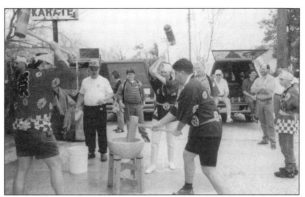

The annual New Year's rice pounding at the Houston Budokan. Pounding rice from left to right are: Ken Kuhlman, Claudia Smith, and Paul Anderson.

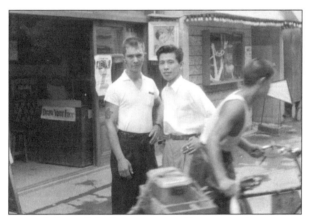

1956 Yshuhiro Takahashi Sensei—Darrell Craig's first karate teacher in Japan, Goju Ryu style.

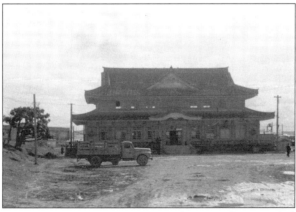

1957 Okinawa—The large gym (dojo) where Darrell Craig studied Shorin Ryu.

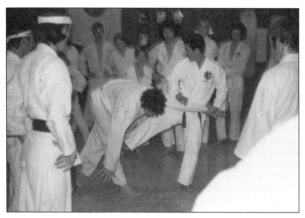

1973 Houston, Texas—at the original Houston Budokan, K. Shorin Sensei demonstrating oyo (the various applications of Piean Yodan).

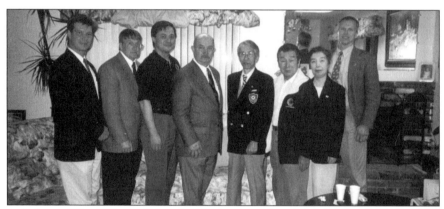

At the home of Kiyoshi Yamazaki Sensei—This photo was taken after joining the All Japan Karate-Do Ryobu-Kai family in 1999. Left to right: Mark Oberkirch, Glenn Ellsworth, Howard High, Darrell Craig, Yakehiro Konishi Sensei, Kiyoshi Yamazaki Sensei, Mrs. Konishi, and Tim Mousel.

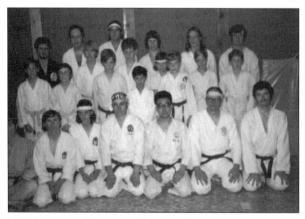

1977 Houston Budokan—T. Oska Sensei during a Goju Ryu clinic (Sensei is sitting in the center of the front row).

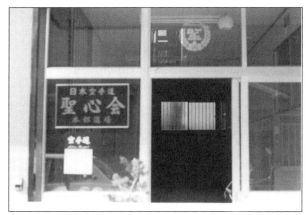

Hombu Dojo for Motobu-ha Shitoh-Ryu Seishin Karate: Osaka, Japan.

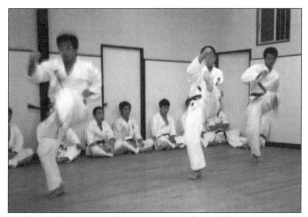

Inside Hombu Dojo, students practicing advanced kata.

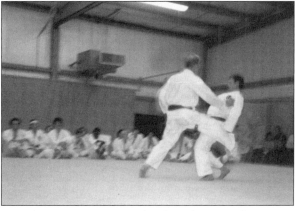

1975 Clinic in Houston, Texas—this photo shows Darrell Craig sparring with K. Siyogo Sensei.

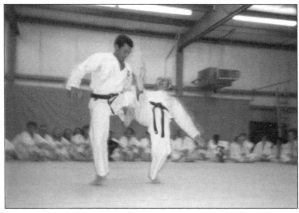

This photo shows what happens when you spar with K. Siyogo Sensei if your attack is too brisk as seen in the previous photograph.

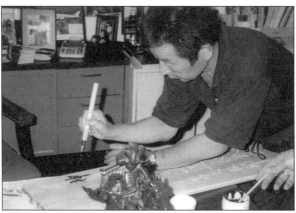

1999—Kiyoshi Yamazaki Sensei making a sudare (authorization sign) for the Houston Budokan Dojo.

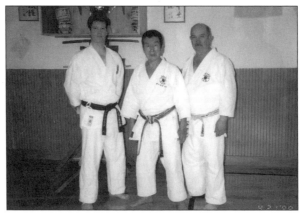

1999—Left to Right: Mark Oberkirch, Kiyoshi Yamazaki, and Darrell Craig at a clinic at the Houston Budokan for Ryobu-Kai students.

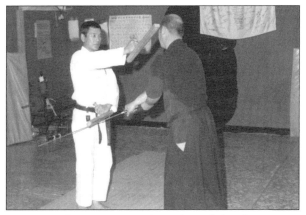

K. Sensei teaching Craig Sensei the Bunkai with the Okinawan tonfa (also called a crutche or guai).

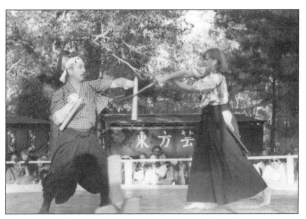

Craig Sensei demonstrating at a Japanese Festival what the master had taught him.

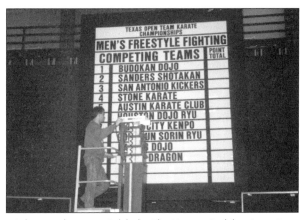

Working on the movie Sidekicks. The Houston Budokan is not in the lineup.

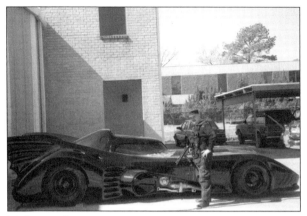

Working on the movie Batman.

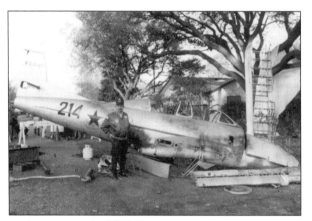

On the movie set of Sidekicks.

CHAPTER TWO

Traditional Kata: The Lost Soul

"Kata is the mother of karate and the bunkai is her soul."
—*Choki Motobu*

"The soul, I fear, has been largely lost."
—*Darrell Craig*

THE SOURCE OF KATA

Kata is said to be the "mother" of karate. Kata are the prearranged and choreographed dance-like forms used in every martial arts style to convey the intricacies of the particular style to the practitioner. In a sense, they are a physical form of oral tradition, a body of knowledge transferring a tradition most historians believe extends from several thousand years ago. Kata are a living record and are not unlike folksongs and dances reverently handed down from generation to generation. They are considered to be the distilled concentrated wisdom, understanding and experience of hundreds of karate masters from centuries of practice. Kata are the basis from which modern day karate techniques have developed and are considered the "textbooks" of the martial arts.

While every martial arts style does kata, few practitioners understand or comprehend their true purpose. The vast majority of karate students just quietly and obediently do kata as part of their instructor's curriculum. To some, kata are viewed as a necessary evil, required to advance on to their next rank. Unfortunately most martial arts students have never been, as one unknown writer said it, "blessed with the inspired tuition of an enlightened teacher, whose solid hand so generously has led to them among a golden path of kata." The richness and beauty of kata have never captured these students' minds and inspired them to practice and perfect these condensed masterpieces of martial secrets and principles.

In order to properly set the stage for the following discussion, we have to go very far back in time and to a very distant place: hundreds of years ago to Okinawa. We could go back even farther, but there's no need to start all the way back at the Fukien Shaolin Temple because the Chinese form of empty-hand fighting, worthy as it is, is a significant step removed from the form it finally took in Okinawa, and then later Japan. So it is in Okinawa that we will start.

Okinawa is an island lying some 750 miles from the Japanese home islands. Centuries ago, the Japanese conquered Okinawa and thus the Okinawans became a people subservient to the Japanese and their culture. After their defeat, the Okinawans were never viewed by the Japanese as their equals. There has been some historical confusion about this. I believe this stems from the word *bushi* that was used by both cultures, although with vastly different meanings. To the Japanese, the word referred to a class of samurai; to the Okinawans, however, it meant someone who had mastered karate kata. Thus, never when referring to an Okinawan did the term signify to the Japanese that the person was of samurai class because there were no Okinawan samurai.

THE SECRECY DEMANDED OF KATA

One of the consequences of their defeat is that the Okinawans were forbidden to possess, much less carry, weapons of any kind. As is frequently the case, this in effect became a cause for further effects. Okinawans, forbidden to possess traditional weapons, developed a system of weaponry using everyday farm implements such as the *sai* (a tool used to turn the soil), the sickle (a tool used to cut grain) and the *tonfa* and *nunchaku* (tools used to grind or crush grain). There were others as well, and they led to the development of a whole weapons system of martial art called *kubodo* which is beyond the scope of this book. Another effect of the prohibition is that it forced the Okinawans to develop a fighting system completely independent of any sort of weaponry, one that relied exclusively on their hands and feet. This, of course, was a huge disadvantage for the unarmed Okinawans who often found themselves in hostile encounters with armed aggressors. Thus, to protect themselves, the Okinawans developed fighting systems for their own private use. The systems were taught within family units, generally at night and in secret. They were closely guarded from outsiders.

The notion of teaching and practicing in secret was not unique to the Okinawans; the same tradition had existed in ancient China. In fact, in ancient China, the masters often had what could be viewed as a dual-track system; they taught the same kata in two slightly different ways. The outer circle of students, those not yet entitled to the master's secrets, would be taught a kata with certain critical details and principles omitted; the inner circle would be taught the same kata, but with those details and principles included. To the untrained eye, the difference might be undetectable. Often the difference involved only forming the hands differently, or attacking at a slightly different angle to reach a different target, or altering the footwork and thereby altering the timing of a particular move. However, the difference was paramount, because the subtle alterations were the difference between a proven, effective waza and one that was only superficially so. Those students who had failed to earn the master's trust, even after years of following in his footsteps, were never admitted into this secret society and thus never became true masters themselves, no matter how much they may have appeared to the untrained eye to be so.

Because the Okinawans were fighting against armed aggressors, the empty-hand systems had to be instantly effective. Subsequently, the systems that developed contained the ability to take a life with one strike. This philosophy, mentioned earlier, became known as *issen-issatsu* or "one strike." The physical ability to take a life with one strike was practiced in waza and keiko; the psychological ability was practiced through kata. It came to be said that, while the Japanese ruled by sword during the day, the Okinawans ruled by fists and feet at night.

The necessity for training in secret from prying Japanese eyes formally ended around 1875 with the withdrawal of the Satsuma Samurai and the recognition that Okinawa was a part of Japan. Thereafter, Okinawan karate began to be identified by specific styles. However, it was not until the early twentieth century that karate became generally known through its introduction as a physical education requirement in the Okinawan public schools. Even though karate was taught in public schools by the early part of this century, it was also still taught within family units in a private setting. In them, much of the tradition of karate was passed on to the younger generation orally. Interestingly, even though the Okinawan culture is over one thousand years old, there is virtually no written history of its fighting systems. This could be due to the great destruction that was visited upon Okinawa in the Second World War. More probably, however, it is due to the fact that, when the Satsuma clan banned weapons in Okinawa for the second time in 1609, the fighting arts had to go underground and be practiced and transmitted to succeeding generations in utmost secrecy. This required that the fighting arts be transmitted orally, and not in writing.

THE ORAL TRADITION OF KARATE KATA

What we know today as Okinawan karate is over a thousand years old. Yet it has no written history. How did this happen? How was an art like karate handed down from generation to generation in secret? The answer lies in kata and the hidden secrets of its bunkai. It also lies in an additional reason that they developed and continued to study this special art. There can be no doubt that the original and primary reason that Okinawa Te was developed and studied was for self-protection. Yet, in time, it became clear to the Okinawan masters that there was an additional, and perhaps deeper, reason to study the art. They realized that the mastery of the bunkai hidden deep within the visible moves of the kata went hand in hand with the mastery of one's self, that discovering the secrets held by the bunkai was secondary to the mastery and perfection of one's own character. This is why the old masters insisted upon the discipline of the kata.

In the late 1920s through the 1930s, there was a famous karate dojo in Tokyo called the Ryobu-Kan. Translated, the name meant "The House of Martial Arts Excellence." The dojo was founded by Yasuhiro Konishi Sensei and Hironishi Ohtsuka Sensei. Initially, the dojo was known primarily for its practice of kata. In time, however, they added *ippon kumite* to the curriculum and it is believed that the techniques for the kumite were taken from the bunkai of their katas. We have always suspected that this decision was largely influenced by Gichin Funikoshi who was teaching karate at Keio University at the same time that Konishi Sensei was teaching kendo and jujitsu there. There was supposedly a sign in the Ryobu-Kan that read "For karate to be perfect, it cannot be just technique, but also education."

Throughout the years, many great Okinawan karate masters visited the Ryobu-Kan. They included Chojun Miyagi (the founder of *goju-ryu*), Kenwa Mabuni (the founder of *shito ryu*) and his student Kosei Kokuba. However, one master stood head and shoulders above the rest, and that was Choki Motobu. He made more defining contributions to the dojo through his knowledge of the katas and their bunkai than anyone else. Motobu Sensei let the primacy of kata be known in the world of karate. In his mind, kata was the mother of karate and the bunkai was her soul. From research and conversations with old senseis, it was discovered that Motobu Sensei taught each kata differently, seeking to draw out a different lesson from each one. For example, he might teach one kata with a method that caused the students to feel heavy in their legs and stomach. For another, he might want the students to feel light, with relaxed shoulders, and perform the kata with agility and speed in quick, linear movements. This type of training was extremely difficult, because it required the students to alter not only their rhythm, but also their feelings and philosophy of each move of each kata. Thus, they had to constantly alter their attitudes regarding the katas as they went from one kata to the next.

The objective of this type of training, which apparently was successful, was to cause the karateka to begin each kata with a fresh mind, enthusiastically yet humble. This type of training also developed in the karateka what the Japanese called *ateru* and *mushin*. *Ateru* is the subconscious development of correct distance, vision, timing and accuracy. This brought one into a state of *mushin*, which means "no mind." I believe that this type of training eliminated the undesirable element of fantasy—or lack of reality—that so often afflicts the martial arts today.

THE TWO SCHOOLS OF KARATE: EXHIBITION AND TRADITIONAL

Today, the practice of karate can be broadly categorized into two schools: on the one hand, we have modern karate for sport. On the other, we have karate as true budo. Generally, the school prevalent in a country depends largely upon the culture and traits of the country in question.

Many of the founders of "modern" martial art styles never trained under a true master. Thus, many never learned the inner teachings of a traditional art. Furthermore, in an attempt to commercialize the art they watered down whatever techniques they did know in order to make them safer to practice. In addition, there is little if any, *okuden* or bunkai in these modern arts because it is no longer necessary to keep techniques secret. Unlike the original purpose of traditional karate, which was combat effectiveness, the main purpose of modern systems is sport or self-expression. The deadly secrets interwoven into the traditional karate katas are contrary to the principles of sport competition that dictate a level playing field for all participants. It is fine for practitioners to choose to "play" karate, but when their competitive days are over, no one should mistake them for karate masters, no matter how many pretty trophies adorn their shelves. In their youth, these people probably had power and strength; when that leaves them, they will have nothing but memories. They will never have developed a real understanding of karate. On the other hand, when the true master reaches that age, he will still have his traditional kata full of wonderful hidden secrets to practice and teach to the next generation.

By virtue of this emphasis on sport, karate and, by extension, kata have been watered down over the years to their least violent denominator that is acceptable for sport practice. The dojos that are responsible for this have opted for commercial success and popularity over the higher goal of preserving a worthy tradition and art. This was brought home most forcefully several years ago when a call from the curator at the Japanese Consulate General's office requesting a karate demonstration at the Houston Children's Museum. During the conversation, the curator mentioned that his ten-year old son was a black belt. "Oh, that's nice, what style does he practice?" "Style? What do you mean style?" was the reply. An explanation began about the major styles of karate when he broke in and said that his son took "Japanese taekwondo." There was a rather pregnant pause after an attempted explanation that taekwondo was a Korean art and that we were going to demonstrate a Japanese art. "What's the difference?" he asked. It was explained that while both employed kicks, punches and strikes, the two originated under different circumstances and, as a consequence, were not exactly alike.

The practice of kata must be taken seriously. True kata performed correctly is kata performed realistically. One must practice kata as though the threat of danger is always there. Once you have practiced long enough, then there is no longer a question; the enemy is always there. Kata trains the mind to look first at what is advancing and respond with the training that has now become subconscious. When someone observes an old sensei, someone who has been practicing kata for many years, they know the practitioner is visualizing many attackers coming at him. Properly done, kata will make the hair on your arms stand up on end.

Kata demonstrates dedication to the martial arts and dedication to kata means seriousness. Kata demonstrates the ability and character to stick to something you said you were going to do, long after the mood you said it in has left you.

The day after our demonstration, which consisted of only kata and the bunkai to one of the katas, the curator called me to complain that our demonstration was far too violent for young children to watch. He then inquired as to why we did not use pads on our hands and feet. I told him that we do not practice our art that way and, as he surely noticed, not one punch or kick actually touched a demonstrator. "Yes", he replied, "but if one had then someone would have been injured." "What do you think karate is all about?" I asked. He said "Obviously I thought I knew, but if your school was demonstrating karate, then I did not have a clue. My son only plays karate, and if I thought he could get hurt doing it I would stop the lessons at once." I suspect this to be the feeling of a lot of parents, because they have been introduced only to the watered down version of the art and not the real thing.

Over the years Craig Sensei attended many karate tournaments, originally as a participant in the kumite and later as the coach of his students or a judge. Over these years, the divergence between the karate as he was taught it (and teaches) and the karate that was being demonstrated became more and more pronounced. This was particularly true in the kata competition. Silly gyrations in colorful costumes set to music bearing no relationship to the series of interwoven, battle-tested techniques that constituted the traditional katas. They appeared to be "mix and match" products of various systems that ended up as an illogical mess based, it would appear, on the mistaken belief that the mixture would produce an end result that was greater than the sum of its parts. It was a sad illustration of a worthy tradition and centuries of painstaking effort being discarded in favor of the novel, the cutting edge, or the worthless.

To be effective, kata training must employ sound, basic techniques combined with advanced combinations that, with proper instruction, the student can eventually understand. Only then will the student be able to defend himself using the techniques found in the kata. The arm-waving, high kicking and other acrobatic foolishness that characterizes modern kata are utterly impractical. The answer continues to lie in the study and practice of the traditional katas. They are boring to the modern student, raised in an age of instant gratification. To the modern student, the traditional katas are not at all what they see in the movies; the katas seem to be just a bunch of down blocks, middle blocks, kicks and lunge punches. The average student will perform these moves hundreds of times and never realize, perhaps because his instructor does not know, the devastating bunkai that just a slight variation of these moves will produce. For example, the average student today does not know the meaning of the statement that "the block is one half of the punch." What it means, and what he would know if he trained under a traditional sensei, is that the block and the punch are inseparable; they are not two separate moves even when performed with the same arm. This means that, in most cases, there is no need to step forward to punch; you block the attack with the forearm and punch with the fist simultaneously.

Frequently at these tournaments I was asked to judge kata. This was very difficult for me because I did not know how to judge the performance of a routine I considered meaningless. I was not alone in this. At one tournament I was talking to an old friend of mine, a man who had grown up in a traditional kung fu environment and was, himself, a teacher of many decades experience. He watched the kata participants and then turned to me and said, "That must be one of your students." I was dumbfounded. It was one of my students, but he had never met him. "How did you know?" I inquired. "Because he is the only one doing a kata that I can understand," was his reply.

Rather than practicing and studying kata for actual functional purposes, too many of today's students do only do kata. They practice only for self-expression, or, stated another way, to "look good." Kata cannot be viewed as a "doing" exercise; it must be viewed as a "using" experience. By this I mean that the student, when performing the various techniques contained in the kata, must employ visualization against an imagined attacker. If, for example, the first move of the particular kata is a middle block followed by a lunge punch, the student must try to visualize the exact angle of the punch that the middle block will deflect. He must try to visualize the exact body position of his attacker. This will enable him to visualize the correct *ma-ai* for his lunge punch as well as visualize the punch hitting the desired vulnerable point on his attacker. Exhibition kata is largely a "doing" exercise. On the other hand, kata performed as a "using" experience is an appraisal tool. If a technique contained in the kata has failed to produce the desired results against an opponent in kumite, careful study of the kata will, in many cases, reveal to the observant student the reason for the failure.

From what I have said, it follows that, in order to do traditional kata correctly, the student must understand the inherent bunkai. This is not to say that the bunkai is revealed when the kata is demonstrated; the whole purpose of the kata in the first instance was to preserve the bunkai in a hidden fashion. But the student must at least know the bunkai. Only from a sensei, who knows and who has a desire to teach the hidden bunkai, will a karateka achieve progress on his road to perfection.

Even though we are now in the twenty-first century, we believe that there are still many people who would like to excel in the martial arts for their original purpose: self-defense and self-improvement. However, when many of today's students begin their martial arts training, they quickly become mesmerized by the belt chase. That is, to achieve the first, and then the next and finally the black belt. Belts—and particularly the black belt— are seen as the ultimate goal and purpose of the study. This is wrong. Students should be made aware of a higher calling. They should use their training to mold their own characters and become better persons. The opponent we should all seek to defeat is within ourselves. Every traditional karate kata begins with a defensive move and in this it is revealed that the art is not designed to foster external aggressiveness. Kata is combat with oneself. The black belt is supposed to be awarded to those students who have expended numerous hours honing their bodies and minds with the discipline that kata demands. It is supposed to symbolize the expert who has learned not only the physical and mental aspects of the art, but also the secrets of the bunkai. The true black belt can sense his opponent's thoughts and anticipate his moves before they occur. He can then react appropriately. He can do this because the true black belt has spent those hours with his kata, and realizes that each of its bunkai is designed to address specific situations. This realization becomes instinctive and the responses automatic. The wearer of a black belt who cannot do this is not a true black belt. He does not possess a deep understanding of the art and has very little to pass on to the next generation of students.

CHAPTER THREE

Some Know Better

"Some know better, some know not. Some care not to know at all and some know and will never say."
—Darrell Max Craig, Sensei.

EVERYTHING IN LIFE IS KATA

Martial arts kata are a set of prearranged movements in which the person doing the kata is engaged in battle with an imaginary opponent. Kata contains all of the movements found in karate and after practicing any, some, or all of these movements hundreds of thousands of times, these movements become embedded in the subconscious of the practitioner. At this level, the movements of kata are as natural and instantly available to the practitioner as any of his other reflexes.

Consider that everything in life is kata. If you do the same thing over and over, that's kata. When you get up in the morning and brush your teeth in a certain way, if you are sitting a table and you put the silverware exactly like you want each and every time, this is kata. Every driver in an Indianapolis 500 race shifts gears thousands of times before the race to know how he should shift, how the car reacts, how it moves; this is kata. Kata is about research and performing to the maximum of one's ability. To do this you have to do movements over and over again. Ballet, tap dance, and race driving are kata. Most people do not see it as kata, but this is what it really is.

Kata is about doing something over and over until it's perfect. This pursuit is, of course, infinite because there is not one thing in life that is perfect. But, those who seek perfection have to make repetition in what they are seeking. This is kata.

THE MODERN TEACHING OF OLD WAYS

A prospective student said to Craig Sensei after observing a kendo (sword arts) class that he had "wanted to do the martial arts like that all of his life." Craig Sensei humbly and quietly replied, "I have."

For a little more than the past fifty years, many things have happened to influence the development of karate. Most significantly is the emergence of a preference to practice mostly sparring and fighting. Westerners, Americans in particular, have always understood and known about fighting. But what they are losing or perhaps have even lost is an understanding of kata's relevance to fighting. This can be traced to the consequences of having a huge population of Westerners spending only a few years in Asia and they never having come to understand why kata is so important.

Even the talent of a natural athlete requires the instruction of a great coach to cultivate and achieve its potential. And like all things, kata degrades over time without a sensei to cultivate it correctly. It is a truism that in all martial arts, not just kata, it takes three things: the student's willingness to learn, a sensei and the sensei's sensei.

In contemporary American society, non-martial artists included, students often do not stay with an informed instructor long enough to gain that teacher's trust. Often true teachers feel that some students are never ready to know the hidden and secret parts of kata. Too often unfortunately, it is the fault of the instructor who just does not know. As a consequence the instructor does not show to the student strikes, the practical techniques or even the more deeply hidden parts.

This happens in the traditional eastern karate disciplines as well. Craig Sensei was discussing things with a class one evening and someone asked, "How long does it take to make a good sensei?" The Sensei said, "Oh perhaps, twenty years." He paused dramatically and then said, "What you really want to know is how long does it take to make a great sensei?" Pausing again, he continued, "I do not know, maybe I won't know until after I am gone."

Craig Sensei's theory and thinking about kata is that learning other kata is like having another wife. He said once, "I got one and one is enough, I do not possibly understand everything there is to understand about this one. Why would I want to get another one?"

Craig Sensei occasionally will rhetorically ask the class, "How long does it take to make a good swordsman? A lifetime. How long does it take to create martial perfection with a pistol or rifle? For some, just a couple of years." Unfortunately today's weapons maximize destruction while minimizing the skill required.

Traditionally and for tens of generations, a sensei or master teacher would not allow students to ask questions about a kata, they would not allow the student to do anything except, as Craig Sensei says, "mimic, movement for movement, step by step, breath by breath, each single movement as they taught it to you." Bunkai is stepping in your sensei's footsteps without question. It is following instruction without question.

But all is not lost. Before you assume that the authors have stepped off of the skeptical cliff of pessimism, we should state that we believe that history is never lost, rewritten yes, but entirely lost forever is rare. The gems and nuggets of teachings in kata are foolproof in that they are designed for a person to dig them out, cut and polish them. This takes time and the need for time is the fundamental conflict existing in our society and culture today. There is not enough time for the student to discover the jewels lying beneath the surface of kata.

BOXERS AND BALLERINAS

Time is a terrific gardener. It weeds out the truly committed and dedicated students. This is how many in the martial arts world explain the fact that traditional martial arts have only a small number of students. For example, a boxing gym will never be overrun with people because when one begins to observe closely the boxers themselves, they look pretty rough and beat up. Observe the ones that have been around along time; they look like it.

If you ever see a prima ballerina's feet, you will be horror stricken. When she gets off of the stage after an exceptional performance, she will take off her pumps and her feet will be bleeding. Like a dedicated martial artist, this is the consequence of the amount of practice and dedication it takes. Like kata though, to the observer, it is just beautiful.

If we consider further the metaphor of a ballerina in the ballet, it exquisitely parallels the performance of kata. In fact, as it was said earlier about all things in life, the ballerina is indeed performing kata herself. Relative to the contraction and expansion, the hard and the soft, of kata, the observation is that no one ever sees a practiced ballerina jump into their partner's arms tense. She performs exactly as a kata should be performed with expansion and contraction of her power, the flow, hard and soft.

There are three principles to kata, principles that can be applied to boxing and ballet: the contraction and expansion of the body, the soft and hard control of power and the proper speed.

The first principle, contraction and expansion of the body, is what ballerinas are exquisite at. If you jump up and spin 360 degrees, you are going to have this one. The other is the soft and hard control of power. If you land too hard you are going to hurt your feet. The proper speed of the technique is critical. Speed is what translates into the grace of making something look easy when it is in fact quite difficult. When a ballerina jumps into the air, or jumps into he arms of a partner, she appears as though she is as light as a feather. Now we know that she is not, but it is the gracefulness of the kata she practices; she knows how to lift, she knows how to present herself, she knows how to look like she is flying.

To one extreme, some people even consider the performance of kata to be effeminate. In our opinion, women *do* possess a seemingly unique and remarkable ability to grasp the more sublime elements of kata. There are many extraordinarily accomplished women, Claudia Smith for example, (see photos), that do kata, and karate in general. Karate would likely benefit from the influence of more women such as Claudia.

In modern martial arts, many students also figure that kata is not important and inferior because the only important and superior use of a students valuable martial time is fighting. Some people do not do kata because it is harmless compared to sparring.

Kata is extraordinarily unique in that it designed to train not only the mind, but the body as well. Kata is not intended just for intellectual self-defense alone; it is equally designed for the movements that train the body. The movements of kata contract and expand the body. Kata teaches how to control power through softening and hardening. Kata teaches the proper speed of techniques and the flowing movements that are needed to make a technique work smoothly.

A vast majority of teachers, instructors, students and scholars today have learned either one or another, kata or fighting. Most of these people, as a general observation, do not know the proper application of the hard and the soft control of power in the kata or understand the correct contraction and expansion of the body. Without proper guidance, it may well be impossible for the student to develop the proper bunkai of kata. If these elements are left out, ignored or left unknown by ignorance, the student cannot ever possibly develop the proper bunkai of kata.

THE CREEPING EFFECT OF NOVICE TEACHERS

Just because a teacher has many certificates hanging on the wall, this does not mean that they are an expert or even a good teacher. Avoid the trap at all costs of an unknowledgeable sensei. Unfortunately, the rapid profusion of the martial arts has made it nearly impossible to avoid this trap of the unknowledgeable sensei today.

There are many teachers and instructors that were never very good competitors. There are many great competitors that make poor teachers. But every once in a while you will run across a great competitor who is also an outstanding teacher or vice versa. An outstanding teacher is one that can teach their students how to break down a kata and discuss its constituents.

An unfortunate degradation has happened with the Americanization of kata. Early on, when karate first came to the United States, karate was like an infant child, and like all children, it wanted to grow up to fast. It is unfortunate that over the last fifty years, when viewed in the context of the thousands of years of karate's history, karate has been taught by orphans who had, at best, absentee parents. American-taught karate rarely had a mother or father because the mother or father remained back in a foreign country.

Practicing for the trick and not working on the technique is one of the reasons that many view American karate culture that is so superficial. In the past, the martial arts have felt the effect of a "watering-down" syndrome. Often, usually right after a student attains first degree black belt, they open their own school and start teaching. They are still just seeds themselves. They have not yet bloomed, and are teaching something that they barely can do themselves. They often make a mistake of believing that since they are clever and read a lot, they can do kata, fill in what they cannot remember and make up the rest.

What has happened to modern kata is that it has been re-adapted so often that there is no depth to the actual teachings themselves. How many students become teachers who have never trained with someone who is really involved in traditional or old-fashioned kata? How many are being taught the bunkai which make the kata truly valuable and powerful. As long as the person does not know the secret of the real kata, the kata is not valuable to them because it has no purpose other than simple punching and blocking. Today's kata is missing the meaning. Too often kata is a meaningless exercise, and while every generation concedes that the old-fashioned, traditional karate kata has faded quite a bit, it is certainly not dying out.

But this is not meant to be as cynical as it sounds; there is much hope for the future. There is a new generation of students now, ones that received their black belts when they were nine or ten and are now in their late twenties and thirties, and really just starting to realize what the martial arts are supposed to be like. They are older and are seeking out the old-fashioned types of martial arts schools because they no longer want the flashy stuff; they have been through that already. More and more, these same students want more depth and knowledge. These maturing students can easily tell in one look or from one lesson whether a school is real or not.

KATA'S STAYING POWER

Kata has staying power because all students eventually realize the futility of reinventing the wheel of an art that has been around for thousands of years. Kata, the mother of karate, has evolved into an almost perfect way of testing oneself to determine one's limits. Students must trust in the fact that there is a lot of experience in the kata that they may not understand. They must understand that there are reason for the way kata has been designed and those reasons have been proven over thousands of years— literally.

The basic foundation is the foundation of Japanese and Okinawan karate itself. This is described in the concept of *ni sente nashi*, a saying by Funikoshi Sensei which translates as, "in karate one does not make the first move." This is to say that all kata begin with a defensive technique, a block. The hidden technique may be entirely mental.

It follows that if someone is instructing you about any kata and that particular kata starts with a punch to the opponent's face, then you can safely suspect that this person does not know what they are doing. Basically, it is not even a kata, it is not even karate, it cannot be because, as Funikoshi said, "all traditional kata start with a block because someone has to attack you for it to work." As soon as a student is given their black belt they want to open their own school. They have forgotten the kata as it was taught to them. These newly minted black-belted instructors must simply make things up, particularly with regard to kata. Consider that a first degree black belt or a second degree black belt would have no credentials to open the school in traditional martial cultures such as those especially found in Japan, Okinawa and China.

What happens when this population of instructors ages? Now this cultural dilemma becomes severely exposed. Today, more than ever, older martial artists are increasingly starting up their own styles that include the developing and creation of its requisite katas. Too often today, the only thing recognizable in kata is perhaps some small part or sequence from an earlier kata by their original teacher. Seeing more than that today is both notable and amazing.

Often a martial arts instructor is measured by the public by the number of kata that they can do. From the traditional martial roots comes the lesson that it is not important how many kata that you do, it is more important to do well the few that you do know.

What too often happens is the changing of a technique because the novice teacher thinks that it would look better with some minor alteration. This creeping effect happens because the instructor feels that he can answer his student's questions better by applying his own interpretation to it. When pressed by inquisitive students asking exactly what are they doing in any particular kata, instantly and often unconsciously the instructor makes something up.

This is an instinct, not good, not bad, just denied.

Today's karate culture, which is reflected in the quality of our kata, is made up of styles developed under the pretenses of, "I am taking the best of the techniques from several other styles, plus a little technical instruction from some karate magazines, as well as some experience from a recent clinic and a couple of tricks from some videos I ordered."

All of a sudden there is a huge population of instructors who are constantly learning all of these moves from all sorts of different styles. They do not, however, understand any of them. "Oh this is a block, " is heard so many times.

LANGUAGE, TRANSLATION, MISINTERPRETATION, AND IGNORANCE

We believe that the explanation of the layered complexity of kata that this book attempts to bring to light is lost in the often poor translations of the various words and descriptions of kata.

In the East, debates about the sophisticated facets of the bunkai of kata have continued for tens of generations. There are certainly more than a few books that have been written in the Japanese, Chinese or Okinawan languages that have never, and may never be translated on this subject alone.

When time has separated the intention of an art from its originators, then only language remains to communicate. At the core, this is the most significant problem in martial culture today. In the translation from one language to another, Japanese or Chinese to English for example, it is often found that not only that words have been inaccurately transcribed but that complete ideas have often been manipulated. Like the 25 Eskimo definitions for snow, the translation of a single word can have so many varied and expressly different meanings.

For example, many people today commonly refer to a living teacher of Japanese martial arts as an "O-sensei." Some even address them this way as in, "Hello, O-Sensei." O-sensei closely translates as "great dead teacher." O means big, ko means little. Well, who's going to round around calling themselves ko-sensei? A little sensei? They want to be an "O" sensei. O-sensei is a Japanese term that, when used colloquially, describes someone who has passed on.

Craig Sensei told a story of knowing a particular gentleman who was a very respectable judo teacher, however he kept calling himself "O-sensei."

He would sign his letters, "O-sensei." And although he was indeed really old, he was also still much too alive to be an O-sensei. Occasionally an astute student or person that speaks the Japanese language would ask how it was possible that an "O-sensei" could be coming to town, they should be passed on and quite unable to travel! To some it was a joke and to others it was a little shameful. Everyone that knew the true intended meaning of O-sensei found this very disrespectful.

Sometimes the interpretation fails altogether. Craig Sensei often told stories about his conversations with Chiba Sensei. "Once," sensei said, " I called my sensei a master. He got very bent out of shape in an instant and he rebuked me sternly. He told me forcefully that I am not a master. And Craig Sensei asked Chiba Sensei, "Well, Sensei are you not my master?" Chiba replied quickly, "No I am not, I am your instructor, perhaps your teacher, but I am no master. My father would have been your master as he was my master." Puzzled Craig Sensei said, "Yes, but Sensei, your father is dead." And he replied confidently, "That's right. And one day I'll be dead. And when this happens I will be there to look over you and then I will be your master. Then I will be your master because, as a master should, I will be in your every breath, I'll be in every breeze, I'll be in every thing that you are, I'll be there for you when you need me. Then perhaps I will be your master, until then, I can only be here in this human body and teach you as our master has taught."

The words bunkai, O-sensei and master are examples of often severe interpretive misunderstanding.

At this point in the book, the authors want to express that it is important to understand, in spite of the serious tone of this book, there are rarely any karateka who maliciously intend to change kata. The changes that have occurred in kata over the past several generations have occurred because it is part ignorance by some instructors and part arrogance by the students.

Craig Sensei once told a story that clearly demonstrated the evolution of a kata. "Years ago one of my students at the school, who is actually a sensei now, went to a tournament in Las Vegas, Nevada. There was an older instructor coming in from Okinawa to teach at the tournament and my student wanted to meet this respected teacher as he had admired him for years. My student wanted to learn a kata by him. Of course, my theory and thinking about kata is that learning another kata is like having another wife. I do not possibly understand everything there is to understand about this one. Why would I want to get another one?"

He continued, "Bunkai required that the only way we were going to be able to bring this particular kata home was to have a strategy. This particular teacher would not allow flash bulbs, pictures, videos…nothing. The strategy was that we would both attend the clinic and my student would learn you learn the second half of the kata and I would learn the first half. When we get back to our room that evening we would put the halves together and see if we could come up with the complete kata. The next day we were having the same clinic again, so we figured that we would be able to check how we were doing with our system."

"It worked, we came back to our own school and we had ourselves a kata, just a kata. Within three months, we lost what ever bunkai of the kata we managed minimally capture." "We changed the foot movement and we changed the hands because we did not have an instructor there to correct us. By our own blundering we slowly changed the position of the feet. Immediately we were no longer even doing the bunkai."

The depth and richness of kata is fleeting to most. Practitioners do not realize what they already know in a kata until they have lost it and paid to learn parts again at a clinic, during a tournament or from a visiting sensei. From years of experience teaching around the country in these types of clinics Craig Sensei has found this to be a recurring theme. From Craig Sensei's perspective, most students at clinics are pleasant to instruct because they are all there as just that, students. They simply have a lessened awareness of the distinction of rank and they are all there because they want to learn, not compete. Classrooms and dojos seem to change this.

But Craig Sensei also says that, for the most part, these very same students and are often dumbfounded when he breaks apart a kata and demonstrates, movement for movement, what exactly they should be doing—the bunkai.

"An awful lot of intelligence can be invested in ignorance when the need for illusion runs deep." (Saul Bellow)

There is a tremendously large population of martial artists out there, particularly North American, who believe that bunkai is the hidden parts of kata, and it is not. There are also those fortunate few, who indeed understand what bunkai truly is, but know very few, if any, katas. Then there are the exceptionally rare few who know what the sacred techniques are in the most intended sense.

The sensei said that, "In my small amount of experience, when I give clinics about kata, I used to want to overwhelm the crowd and impress them with the knowledge I knew the students and observers really did not know. However, in time and with experience, I quit teaching this way because I would unintentionally embarrass people, occasionally other good instructors who were very well known and whose kata was beautiful.

Unfortunately, even good instructors, when shown the bunkai, the oyo or the kakushi, understood it strictly as bunkai. They would rarely admit that they did not really know the difference."

Now I do not wish to seem hypocritical, but the reader has to understand that sometimes a block is executed exactly as the original teacher taught it. Then this is bunkai, accidental or not. If you say it is a block, and it looks like a block, it is probably bunkai. If you say it is a kick and it looks like a kick and it is to the mid section or some such target, in most cases a target is where you have bunkai.

The pattern is that, when pressed, kata students will often refer to the differences in "their" kata and "your" kata even among those in the same style. They will say, "well, we do it almost exactly like that." It is futile to tell them that they are not actually doing the bunkai. In most cases, an entirely self-made up kata is in fact kata, but it cannot be bunkai. Some styles insist that students do made up kata for rank tests. There can be found little or no recognizable bunkai. Often they just demonstrate a profound misunderstanding of bunkai.

Today, unfortunately, most martial artists, as students, are not ready to absorb the true complexity and depth that most kata have to offer. As a consequence, we have evolved away from understanding the various layers and toward the superficial display of meaningless entertainment.

Kata is a language of symbols. Kata itself is a non-verbal form of communication whose meaning cannot be realized through words or images. In order to be communicated, kata must be done, not written, not spoken, not even read about.

BUNKAI, OYO, HENKA AND KAKUSHI

Kakushi is something that the student may never discover or know. While researching this book, Craig Sensei once casually said something that succinctly demonstrates the sophistication of kata. He said casually; "There are a lot of katas I do that I do not know the hidden parts to. Now, some kata I know the hidden part because I know the hidden part from another kata and it is the same technique and moves. But even with my years of experience and learning from very knowledgeable teachers themselves, there are kakushi that will never be known."

Bunkai is what gives kata its purpose. However, bunkai is often very loosely translated into meaning something about the hidden techniques within kata. When you talk about the hidden techniques, this is where we have developed the misunderstandings about bunkai. People consistently define bunkai as being the hidden part or parts to a kata, no bunkai is the visual part. Bunkai is the part that an observer or spectator can actually see when the kata is being performed.

There was an article in one of the popular budo newspapers that was discussing sword testing. One gentleman was vociferously complaining that another gentleman was indiscriminately leaving out specific single syllables as he was describing test cutting. According to the dictionary perhaps there was indeed a difference between meaning and interpretation. In this instance, they were both right. Unfortunately, the one that he was criticizing had many more followers than the other did. And so if the word is not translated exactly as intended such as with bunkai or oyo, unintended consequences occur.

We have manifested a martial arts culture today that has basically bastardized the interpretation of many words and meanings over time. This is not done through malice; it is mostly done through ignorance. The definition of bunkai, like the other layers of kata, is hidden in the fundamental misunderstanding and mistranslations of the words themselves. The concepts behind the teaching and learning of kata create for a rather confusing subject because we are using as many as four Japanese words to describe and define an idea that we would likely agree that English has no words for. In the context of this book, not only has the idea of bunkai been grossly mistranslated, but we ignorantly and often use it to cover three other profound tenets of kata: the oyo, henka and kakushi. This book, *Shihan Te, The Bunkai of Kata*, is about these four elements of kata.

Craig Sensei told a story about the difficulties of realizing how little we actually know about the bunkai of kata, much less about the henka, kakushi, and oyo. Sensei explained; "I was doing one particular kata for ten years and there was one move in particular that I thought was a really cool. One time someone said to me that what I was actually doing was a technique for stepping over rice paddies."

"I remember asking an American instructor many years ago when we did this stepping move, 'what are we were doing when we were stepping like this?' He said, 'Well, my teacher told me that this technique was for stepping over rice paddies and kicking somebody in the chest.' And so, like every trusting and believing good student I said, 'that sounds good to me.' I of course knew that there were rice paddies in the Orient, so stepping over rice paddies made sense to me."

Sometime later, as Craig Sensei says, " I lost my hair and grew some brains". A Chinese friend of his, an excellent teacher himself said, "You know, Sensei, I have always liked that particular stepping move you do." Craig Sensei, thinking to himself said, "what move is he talking about?"

The friend continued, adding that he thought that that particular move is one of the best moves in all of kata. Inside, Craig Sensei was beginning to wonder why stepping over rice paddies would be a considered a "cool move." Rice paddies? When would one ever be going to be stepping over rice paddies? The fact is that Craig Sensei had wondered about what use it would be to step over rice paddies anyway?

The gentleman kept on referring to that particular stepping move and saying that it "is such a great move. I learned it while I was a kid in China." Then he asked Craig Sensei if he knew and understood what the application of this particular move was. He asked if Craig Sensei knew the oyo.

Craig Sensei thought to himself, "Oh, here we go." Craig Sensei said, "Oh yes, the bunkai, the working parts of the kata." His friend replied, "Yes, the bunkai."

Here is the point of that exchange. Craig Sensei was saying bunkai and his friend was agreeing with him, specifically in regard to the "working part". The failure in translation happening between Craig Sensei's friend (being Asian) and Craig Sensei (being an American) is very apparent here. He was accepting Craig Sensei's incorrect translation of bunkai as meaning the working part.

It turns out that the hidden true, mostly unknown technique of this particular stepping over technique that the Chinese friend admired is a take down, a capture of the attacker's leg and a kick to the groin. Craig Sensei said he quickly confessed that all this time he had believed that the technique was for stepping over a rice paddy and kicking somebody in the knee. Here Craig Sensei had been doing a "hidden" technique all along and believing the entire time that this was absolutely nothing more than stepping over a rice paddy and kicking.

"Was I embarrassed? Oh yes I was embarrassed," Craig Sensei said frankly, "And indeed I did what most other instructors do and faked the application all along. My first thought was that I am not going to embarrass myself by saying that I did not even know what he was talking about," Craig Sensei quietly revealed that "the truth is that, until admitted by a very experienced sensei, that there is no part to this particular kata where one is actually stepping over the rice paddies, it would have always remained obscured to me. Someone who taught me the kata made that up, an American attempting to create an explanation in the absence of the truth." And so, looking back at this whole experience now, Craig Sensei explained that, "the entire time, I was claiming that stepping over rice paddies was the hidden technique. It was not the hidden technique, stepping over the rice paddies represents the bunkai. Because doing the technique was exactly like the kata."

This story perhaps best demonstrates the purpose of this book.

More often than not, today advanced and sophisticated kata are nothing more than the amalgamated parts of other kata welded together to create even more advanced moves. In this case you may not interpret the exact hidden part in the kata as it has always been there, but you may have already interpreted some of the hidden part that is elsewhere in the particular kata.

Craig Sensei had an ideal story to illustrate this observation. "There is a kata in judo called Ju no kata and it is a kata developed by Dr. Jiro Kano, the founder of judo for women. Claudia Smith and I went to a clinic once where we observed someone teaching this particular kata. The teacher was busy explaining each of the various bunkai to this particular kata, but he was not truly explaining the bunkai to the kata, he was actually demonstrating the henka, his own interpretation of what the kata was. He was consistently using the word bunkai because that is the only word that is written down in most books and mostly in reference to the hidden part, but was not a hidden part at all it turns out.

At the time, Ms. Smith was being taught by one of the finest and highest ranking judoka in the world, Fukuda Sensei from San Francisco. Fukuda Sensei was a direct student of Dr. Jiro Kano. In fact, it was her grandfather that taught Dr. Kano the art of jujitsu some one hundred years ago. Sensei continued, "And so I said to Claudia, the next time, just out of curiosity, when you go out to San Francisco and practice, ask her about all the bunkai we saw for this particular judo-kata. It was not that we truly doubted this instructor and we certainly do not believe that there was any malicious intent here, just perhaps some ignorance. But then again, we thought, maybe Fukuda Sensei knows something we do not know. So Ms. Smith was going to take advantage of her next opportunity to talk to Fukuda Sensei about this kata; if there is bunkai, oyo, henka and kakushi to this kata. Were there, in fact, any hidden techniques in this kata as claimed by this particular instructor.

Several months later Ms. Smith went to San Francisco and asked Fukuda Sensei about this. Fukuda Sensei laughed heartily. She told Claudia that she had never heard of such a thing in her whole life about that particular kata. At one point, Ms. Smith showed the sensei one of the so-called ("bunkai") hidden techniques and Fukuda Sensei immediately exclaimed, "Oh! Who made that up?" The fact is that, in this particular judo kata, there is absolutely no hidden moves in it what so ever. This particular judo kata was designed entirely for stretching and exercise. It is essentially a kata not of self-defense, but strictly one of style. That there were so many "bunkai" at all was what was amazing.

It is easy to see how this happens today. Unfortunately, any martial arts clinic invitation that beckons with "come learn the stuff I have made up" would fail to attract any students. However, the one that says, "come learn the bunkai, the hidden, the secret techniques" attracts a multitude of students and sells many tapes and clinics. Unfortunately the yearning student often only pays good money to really learn the made-up parts. This mostly sells into the quick learn mentality of contemporary martial arts and is completely antithetical to the idea that kata takes a lifetime to master.

Zanshin Finishing With Attention

The authors were discussing kata one evening after a particularly long and vigorous class of kendo kata. Craig Sensei said to Paul that, "My first real light bulb of knowledge about karate kata came to me from practicing kendo kata. In the kendo kata I learned from O-Chiba Sensei, I was introduced to the concept and idea of zanshin."

All kata ends with *zanshin*, the mental awareness that lies at the end of a technique. Keep in mind that the hidden techniques found in kata do not always have to be physical. Zanshin is to maintain awareness after completion of a technique or kata. Zanshin is to have a perfect finish and attention to one's last movement.

Craig Sensei continued, "You must absolutely have zanshin to finish a technique. But when I would ask O-Sensei, 'Where is the zanshin in this kata?' He would say, 'In the hidden technique is the zanshin.' And at first, like all bad students, I would say oh yes, I understand, but I really had no idea what he was talking about. None—zero. Please do not make the mistaken assumption that O-Sensei did not know the secret techniques, he most certainly did. However, what happened here was that, because I did not know any better, he did not show it to me, but he indeed answered my question completely."

With regard to American karate culture, one might rightly ask if we have we lost the truly secret intended techniques? Does anybody actually know or even teach these secrets anymore? Did they ever? The answer, certainly, is still yes.

SEE THE LIGHT OR FEEL THE HEAT

Some people change when they see the light. Some people change when they feel the heat. Some people require blunt force trauma.

> *Neo: "Why do my eyes hurt?"*
> *Morpheous: "Because you have never used them before."*
> —The Matrix, *1999, Warner Brothers.*

All forms of kata are indeed complex and sophisticated. So complicated and sophisticated at their core that learning from kata can be nearly fathomless. But at the same time, kata is accessible to everyone, regardless of age, condition or stature.

Unfortunately, there comes a point for many who dive into the ocean of the martial arts when they find that they can only swim so deep. The realities of contemporary society limit the ability of most people to dive to the depth of their abilities. Not knowing what lies at the depths below, students, unintentionally masquerading as teachers, create and concoct. With no time to give, the practical secrets of fishing get retold as useless stories of sea monsters.

Fundamentally most martial students today are simply not capable of receiving all of the information that truly exists below the surface of their respective martial arts. Human nature drives the tendency of anybody that is asked a question to err with the indication that they understand, when, in fact, they do not.

Kata was brilliantly designed and intended to be simple and effective way to pass and transmit information from generation to generation. Bunkai is a practical and functional necessity of all kata. The definition of bunkai is simple although many reputations and years of learning may be wrapped up in what it does not mean.

Today in the martial arts, we strive less to pass on the knowledge gained from previous generations and we seem to strive more to create, redesign, modify and change kata to amaze judges and entertain audiences.

One of the expectations of the authors is that some people, perhaps many, will criticize the nature of this book. We implore the reader not to mix the metaphors with the message. The intention here is not to superficially create a point around the confusing semantics of Eastern and Western languages.

At this point, if you believe that the authors intended to teach this particular kata, or introduce this particular style, then you may have or have missed the message of this book, the authors, or both.

We do not believe that we are changing the record as much as we believe that we are setting it straight. The authors' goal with this book is to make the martial artist think, contemplate and consider that language is only one of many challenges in discovering the depths of kata.

In the next chapter, we will certainly explore and strive to clarify what the word and concept of *bunkai* means exactly. It is with our own small effort that we move in the direction of this simple, but radical definition. For clarity's sake here, it is important that our readers understand that we absolutely do not believe we are describing something negative here.

Kata changes for many reasons, some known, and some unknown. These written observations, commentary and explanations are not meant to be critical to change, but to be merely enlightening us that change is happening.

We know little about the pre-European time in American history and this was as recent as 250 years, possibly 500 years ago. The same context applies here to the kata of any martial art. The lack of knowledge arises because many of the secrets, the true interpretations and learning, have been lost. The lineage of Eastern martial arts has evolved for thousands of years. As a consequence, the majority of kata teachings today has become corrupted and bear little resemblance to their origins from as recently as several generations ago.

It is our hope that this book not be read as an attempt to define martial ignorance, but rather be considered a worthy contribution to increasing the awareness outside of what tradition is and the importance of understanding the several purposes and many layers of kata.

This is what this book is all about, letting the reader discover something that maybe they have not seen before. This book is meant to open the eyes of all of those karate students and people out there, and to let them know that there is plenty more to learn within your own katas. You will find, however, that the beauty of kata is to be found in the hardest place to find—that place is within yourself.

CHAPTER FOUR

The Four Elements of Kata: Bunkai, Oyo, Henka, Kakushi

Like the some 25 varied definitions of snow by Eskimo, the basket of kata is woven of the four elements of *bunkai*, *oyo*, *henka* and *kakushi*. These elements are so firmly woven together as a basket that is solid and immovable, but at the same time the basket can be disassembled. Unless you are skilled and practiced like a weaver, once the basket is pulled apart, it can never be put back together. The skilled, practiced weaver, however, can take the basket entirely apart and put it back together repeatedly, each weave becoming tighter and more beautiful than the previous.

BUNKAI, THE FIRST ELEMENT

Bunkai is a word that is overused and probably more misunderstood than any word in the lexicon of the karate. Most people interpret the word bunkai as the meaning of the separate and individual movements performed in the kata. This is only partly correct. Unfortunately, today the word bunkai, because it is the only word we used and is used, utterly fails to capture the breadth and depth of kata.

The definition of bunkai, more clearly stated means the breakdown and analysis of the kata movement, *without any variation of the movements*, as the kata was originally taught. "As taught by the original instructor" is precisely where most of the misunderstandings about martial katas take place because most martial arts practitioners have never been introduced to, much less contemplated, the concept of no-changedness in kata. In the absence of having the ideas of oyo, henka and kakushi attached to kata, bunkai has evolved into a catchall term most often used to describe the hidden techniques of kata. This is not what bunkai was intended to describe.

The traditional approach to teaching the richness of kata is by having the teacher break down the techniques in any particular kata precisely as taught to him (the bunkai). If your teacher shows you a technique from a specific kata, and you learn it exactly as it was shown, and then in you in turn teach that particular technique to your student exactly as it was taught to you, this student then becomes a teacher and he shows it to his student exactly as he was taught, you will have bunkai.

Bunkai, in its more ideal definition, cannot deviate and should remain unchanged from the way the kata was originally taught. This goes to the point where the old-time instructors would not allow you to ever discuss the kata with anyone outside of the sensei's closest circle of students. The sensei's instructors would not allow students to ask questions about the kata; they would not allow the student to do anything except mimic, movement for movement, step by step, breath by breath, each single movement as they taught it to you. Deviation, or to be more precise non-deviation, was carefully controlled by the traditional sensei and schools (ryu).

When the sensei discusses the bunkai as a breakdown of the kata as it was taught, without variation, this is not to suggest that all modern katas are corrupt or superficial in their original intentions. Most people accept the word bunkai as what they see the kata to be, whether it has been explained by their instructor, explained by someone else or interpreted by their own training into something they believe could be potentially used as a self-defense application. This interpretation, often subtle at first, is where many martial arts practitioners begin to create and make things up that are not really there and were never there. This deviation, although not considered to be bunkai, would be considered the idea of *oyo*.

This deviation could also be considered something that is not exactly like the original kata but was created by the practitioner to satisfy a question or to satisfy a physically required movement such as reaction to an injury or particular body type. This is not considered the appropriate application of the idea behind the word bunkai.

In the traditional sense of bunkai, and in fact martial arts, the student basically becomes a puppet, a robot because kata was taught through the absolute mimicking of the movements of the instructor. And here again we, students and teachers alike, have become unfamiliar with the difference between the ideas of bunkai and oyo.

One of the areas where students, teachers and most all practitioners of kata develop a fair amount of misunderstanding is in believing that when kata is performed alone, it is bunkai; and that when it is performed with a practice partner, it is oyo. Obviously this is not the case.

OYO, THE SECOND ELEMENT

Here is an example of bunkai: saying Darrell Max Craig, which is the name as it appears on the cover of this book, is bunkai. If the reader were to say "Darrell Craig" as in, "His name is Darrell Craig," this is oyo. If the reader were to say, "Craig Sensei," that would be henka. However, in all of the previous works written by Darrell Craig, he has never revealed that the hidden part of his name is Max Craig. This was the name of Darrell's father. The hidden part of the name is the word Max. His name, like kata, is as Craig Sensei says, "all of these things."

Craig Sensei explained that, "the reason my name is on the book cover as 'Darrell Max Craig' is because I wanted to honor my father. Perhaps this is an 'unwestern' perspective, but that's my business. That's the secret part, the kakushi and my heart. The corollary here between the way I present my name and the bunkai of kata is that in both cases, the student must read deeper and for a longer period of time to have the secrets revealed."

When somebody says Darrell Max "He's So Serious" Craig, this is henka. This is not anywhere near what the original was, in this case Darrell Max Craig. In fact by saying "Darrell Max 'He's So Serious' Craig" you are, in effect placing a judgment on the technique or kata of Darrell Max Craig. However, just because this an interpretation, specifically yours, this is not to be taken as meaning a bad thing or misinterpreted, it is just not the bunkai. People who do not remember Darrell Craig's first name will instinctively call him, "Craig Sensei". This is not bunkai.

If the reader were to take this book and copy it word for word, he would be doing bunkai. But if you take a copy of this book to a printer and ask him to reproduce this book, you would really not have anywhere near the actual bunkai of kata. What you have is a path through those words you are reading.

It is our hope and intention that anyone reading this book confidently understands that to modify anything from the original movement of a kata is the idea and concept described by the word oyo. Regardless of the kata you are doing, you may, at any moment, actually be doing any one of several things, including not-doing bunkai. You may now, hopefully, realize that it is not a bunkai, that it may in fact be oyo. Or, rather, may not be oyo, it may be henka, and at least two times in this book we will show the kakushi, a hidden technique. Some unique students of the martial arts will find some of these hidden techniques in their own katas, mostly through sheer persistence.

When a sentence is repeated and you understand it well enough to duplicate it, then you have bunkai. Then suppose you added a word into the sentence. Instantly, you get a different kind of meaning. A noun, an adjective, a verb, anything will create a different meaning, an oyo. But do not neglect to remember what the original sentence was—it was the bunkai. Most people forget what the sentence was because it is easier to understand as oyo, the derivative.

The first two things to be understood about kata are the bunkai and the oyo. The first, bunkai, means that there is absolutely no change in the form of the kata, from performance to performance, repetition after repetition. When the practitioner finds himself changing or modifying the kata to make a particular technique work, or make it more "realistic", this is oyo.

In the early history of American karate a certain falsification in the understanding of oyo occurred. Today it would be safe to say that oyo is probably what most instructors and teachers are calling bunkai.

While teaching about kata in clinics and seminars, Craig Sensei will ask a student, "Why are you doing this block?" Typically, a handful of students will politely, respectfully and with the best of intentions say; "oh, this is a twisting knife-hand carotid strike, this is the bunkai." What the student does not realize is that what they are doing cannot possibly be bunkai because at most, it is one or two generations old.

Craig Sensei will generally suggest to the student "it is not technically bunkai, it is something called oyo." There is a pretty common blank stare that begins right about then. For an even better 'deer in the headlights effect,' try to explain henka and kakushi.

The practical application of techniques in kata are usually brought to light in two ways: most often it is through a teacher's instruction in oyo though from time to time a student will uncover it himself. If a student uncovers a practical technique, it is likely not going to be exactly the same oyo as his instructor.

Now let's suppose that your traditional teacher attempts to teach you and you indeed learn the technique exactly as he taught you. You now go to teach it to your student only you have forgotten just a little and you indeed teach it a little bit differently. You no longer have bunkai—you have oyo.

From the traditional understanding of what kata is about and intended for, it is not too rigid to say that a kata must be performed from beginning to end, as originally taught, for it to maintain its bunkai'ed-ness. Again if you vary the application of the movement as originally taught in any fashion or form, you do not have bunkai. You have oyo.

HENKA, THE THIRD ELEMENT

Bunkai is often interpreted as to disassemble, to take apart. It means to precisely take apart, step by step, piece by piece. For example, there is only one way you can disassemble and reassemble an engine. This is bunkai. Performing bunkai on an engine is so essential that when completed, the engine will either run, or it will not. You do the bunkai, without knowing why, exactly because you will know the end result.

If one were to add a supercharger to this engine, this would be oyo. If one were to add a simple chrome muffler, a component that does not functionally change a thing, this would be considered *henka*. Henka defines your interpretation of how you want the engine to look.

It has nothing to do with the actually running of the engine. *Kakushi*, in this automobile analogy, is about what the engine is to be used for, the real purpose; the kakushi would pull a boat trailer.

KAKUSHI, THE FOURTH ELEMENT

In contrast to the novice teacher from the previous chapter, the knowledgeable teacher would then demonstrate these same techniques with an opponent showing each movement as bunkai, oyo, henka—or none at all as Fukuda Sensei explained. If the student were fortunate enough, the kakushi, the truly secret meaning might be revealed as well. Unfortunately, most instructors, but not all, are incapable of teaching to this depth and the education process is flawed from the beginning as one, two or more of the other four elements of kata are left out of the teaching process. Most of the time one will find that an instructor has taught a little oyo and henka, but hardly ever bunkai, except for the initial block. It is extraordinarily rare that kakushi is known, much less shown.

Craig Sensei told a story of a particular time when there were a handful of black-belt students visiting after practice in the sensei's dressing room. The discussion was about and around the very nature of kata that this book explores. The sensei described how he went from junior to senior student, each of whom had been with the sensei as students seven, eight years or more and, asked them what did they think bunkai was? He asked them to give him their explanation of bunkai. Craig Sensei continued, "I received as many different interpretations as there were students sitting there. I then realized although I had been instructing them for many years, that even I had not gotten across to them the difference between the bunkai and the oyo, and much less about the other various layers and shades of kata." Almost apologetically he continued, "I took it upon myself to assume that my students really understood. I have never really explained in depth the distinctions found in kata." This is what is really important about this book.

CAPTURING THE INTENDED SENSE

The challenge today is capturing bunkai in its intended sense. This requires going back to the source, the kata; kata is the mother, the bunkai is the child. Everything flows on from the bunkai. Henka and oyo are the grown-ups, if you will. Kakushi is the master. Mastery takes a long time to achieve, if ever achieved at all. In some cases mastery is impossible to achieve because it has lost.

This is also what the beauty of kata is all about. It is about trying to make the individual stumble and fall, pick himself or herself up, and then find the hidden technique or techniques within the kata itself. A powerful and profound lesson about the essence of kata, in fact karate in general, can be learned from the old Chinese proverb "seven times fall down, eight times get up."

What would a knowledgeable sensei say to a student that came and asked, "Sensei, would you please teach me the kakushi to this kata?" A knowledgeable sensei would probably ask first to see his kata. And, after examining his kata, he would ask to see the student's bunkai. Then he may ask the student to see the their oyo and the henka of any one particular technique. At this point the student would likely be so confused, it would be apparent that he had been genuinely poorly instructed.

The sensei would not use the word kakushi, he would likely say "the hidden technique." The sensei would be satisfied with showing the student just the bunkai—the exact duplicate of what he was taught. Unfortunately then this same student continues on to teach his students oyo, because he cannot remember the exact kata. This is where the confusion is perpetuated.

If you were to kick the knee, the groin, the chest, the pelvis, the solar plexus or the throat, and these movements are from a kata, then this may likely be bunkai. Flying side kicks to the forehead, and double whapper kicks, and aerial-spinning 380-degree kicks that are not feasible most likely are not bunkai. Many can identify the source of a particular kata. In fact, if it is a fairly high kick, it may likely be an Okinawan kata, perhaps Japanese or Korean. Many of the Chinese kicks are low, to the pelvis, and are equally massively disabling.

There is a move in one particularly advanced kata where the practitioner does a 360-degree jumping spin, drops to his feet, blocks and punches. He jumps straight up in the air enough to turn around 360 degrees, land in *kubadachi*, a horse stance, block and punch.

Craig Sensei related a story about the time he once saw somebody performing this technique while doing kata. When Craig Sensei asked what it was they thought that they were doing, they replied, "looking around." A little surprised, Craig Sensei said, "excuse me, you are looking around?" "Yes", came the reply, "the bunkai is that you spin up in the air and while rotating 360 degrees, look around for any more enemies." That was his explanation of the bunkai of this kata.

Unfortunately the true explanation of the bunkai, like Fukuda Sensei stretching kata, is that the 360-degree spin is an exercise for developing balance and coordination. It is extremely doubtful that in a real fight one might find wisdom in jumping up and executing a 360-degree spin—but everybody should try it sometime. Get into a horse stance on top of a sheet of butcher paper, or use tape on the floor and mark around your feet. Now jump a 360-degree spin and try to land in the same foot prints that you put down. See how long it takes you. It's an art, that's why they call it martial arts.

At a tournament at which Craig Sensei was a judge, a competitor stood and announced the name of the kata he was going to perform. Specifically what he said was, "I am going to do one-third of kata A and one-third of kata B and one-fourth of kata C." Right there on the spot he was making up a kata comprised of techniques taken from various other kata. He was demonstrating techniques and movements he quickly threw together only because he thought they were flashy enough to earn him a trophy.

The funny part about this story is that this particular competitor tied for first place. The sensei, as head judge, ruled that this person would have to repeat the kata they had just performed a few minutes before. The competitor replied to the sensei, "I cannot." The sensei said, "What do you mean, you cannot?" He said, "I just made this kata up and I cannot duplicate it exactly. I can get close to it, but I cannot do the exact thing over again." The sensei said, "Then you are disqualified. You must perform the same kata exactly as you just did it or it cannot be kata." In this case the performer of the kata clearly did not understand what bunkai was.

If you follow in the footsteps of your teacher, step by step, never varying from your teacher's footpath, making no side trips or diversions whatsoever, not looking to the right, or looking to the left, only looking into your teacher's footprints so that you can put your foot exactly in his, then you are doing bunkai. If you were to sit down on the side of the road where your teacher did not sit down, you are doing oyo. If you step off of the road and wonder off on down a path someplace looking at the flowers, you are doing henka. And if all you ever do is henka, wandering around, you are eventually going to get lost.

CHAPTER FIVE

Demonstrating the Four Elements of a Kata

If you have been studying the martial arts for any length of time and you have run across some of this kata, part of this kata or all of this kata, it has likely been changed a little bit to fit your Korean style, your Japanese style, or your Chinese style, your Kenpo style. And within any of the traditional world's styles lie those techniques that have always been there for generations upon generations, hundreds of years. The bunkai has changed and been lost because the oyo and henka have crept in and taken over. And kakushi? Kakushi has never and may never be found in any of the katas with the exception of those who have been blessed to have studied under a true master for many decades. The depth of teaching required to discover kakushi is extraordinarily rare in the world, it is rare in Japan, it is even more rare in Okinawa, and it is rare in China.

In the rest of this chapter, we will look at and discuss Figures 1 through 82, and correlate these figures with the four elements of katas discussed in chapter four.

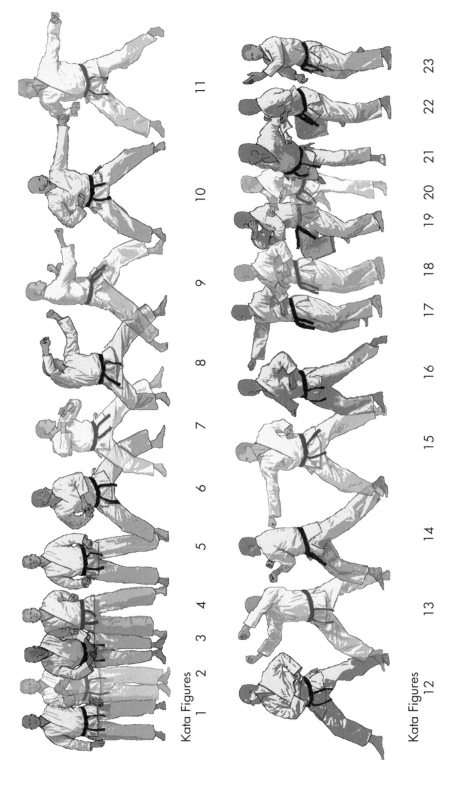

Kata Figures
1 2 3 4 5 6 7 8 9 10 11

Kata Figures
12 13 14 15 16 17 18 19 20 21 22 23

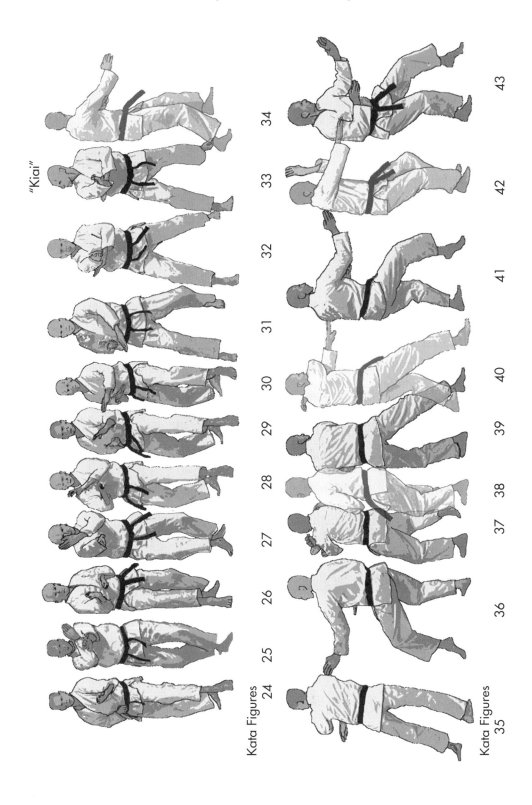

"Kiai"

Kata Figures
24 25 26 27 28 29 30 31 32 33 34

Kata Figures
35 36 37 38 39 40 41 42 43

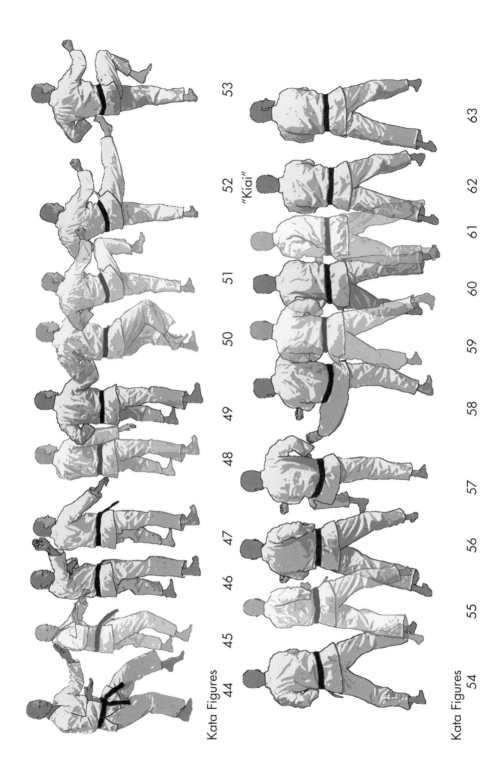

Kata Figures
44 45 46 47 48 49 50 51 52 53
"Kiai"

Kata Figures
54 55 56 57 58 59 60 61 62 63

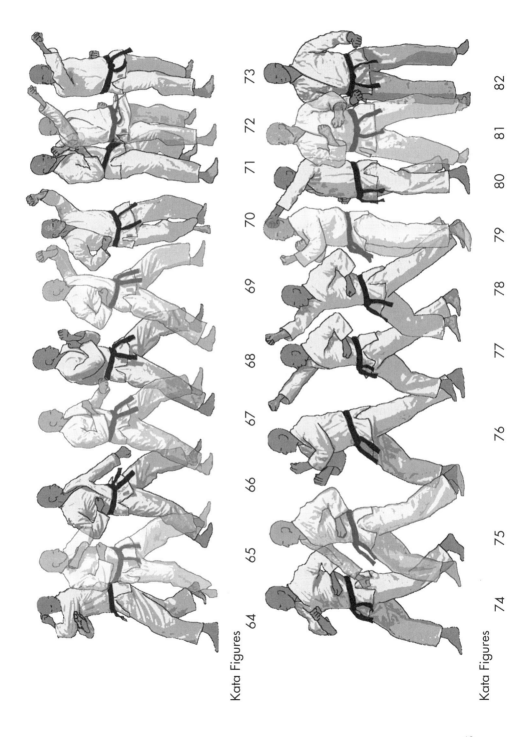

Kata Figures

Kata Figures

DEMONSTRATING BUNKAI

In this particular kata, the initial block in Kata Figure 36 is a knife-hand block from a cat stance. That's bunkai. If you do not take the kata any further than that, then the bunkai is the block.

If you observe the illustrations of the kata, specifically Kata Figures 30 through 33, you can see there is a push block, a pushing down as shown in Kata Figures 30, 31 and 32. Before the person turns their head to look, they have actually finished by Kata Figure 33. The bunkai is with Kata Figures 30, 31 and 32. Because looking at the application in Figures 1, 2 and 3, we have push block; he is using the kata right here in Figure 1, a knife-hand block. Then he pushes down. Now, the question for the reader is if in Figure 2, looking at it very carefully, is he doing bunkai or oyo?

Kata Figures

"Kiai"

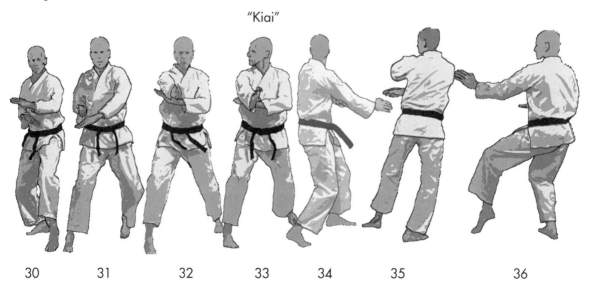

| 30 | 31 | 32 | 33 | 34 | 35 | 36 |

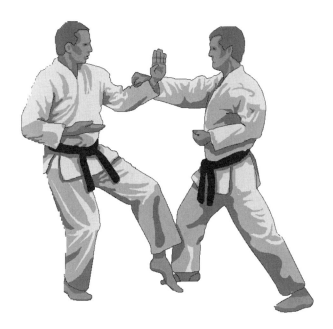

Figure 1

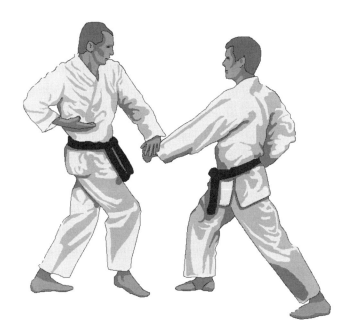

Figure 2

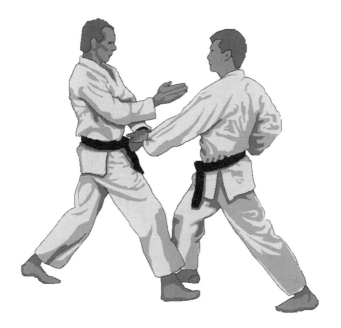

Figure 3

DEMONSTRATING OYO

New problems arise when we begin discussing if oyo is open for interpretation by the student. The answer generally depends on the level and proficiency of the student. The word, or rather the concept of oyo, is a derivative of the traditional intention. For instance, if the reader considers Figure 5, he will find that what is being done is exactly the same as in Kata Figure 8. This is bunkai. Once you go to Figure 6, which is also Kata Figure 9, this is where the practitioner deviates from the bunkai. When we reach Figure 7, we no longer have bunkai because what the person is doing in Figure 7 is not what they are actually doing in Kata Figure 9. Figure 7 is oyo.

Kata Figures

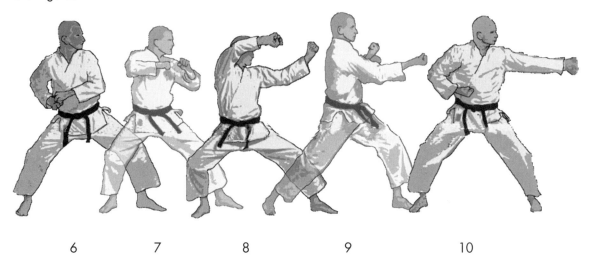

| 6 | 7 | 8 | 9 | 10 |

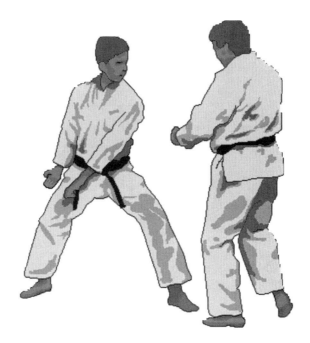

Figure 4

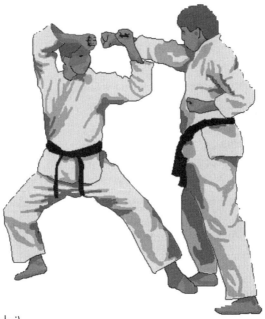

Figure 5 (This is bunkai)

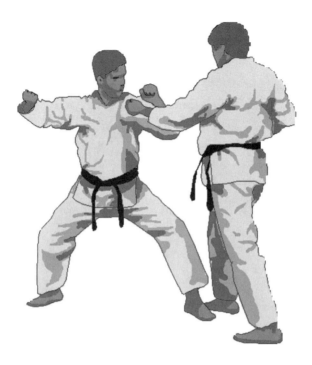

Figure 6

Now if we go back and consider that Figure 7 is oyo, then what should we consider Kata Figure 9? If you are truly doing the bunkai to Kata Figure 9, you will not capture your attackers arm as shown in Figure 7. Instead you will allow the attack to slide by your right ear. The block will happen at the same elevation as the right ear and you will immediately go to the position demonstrated in Kata Figure 10 punching the opponent in the throat. This would be considered the bunkai. However, in Figures 7 and 8 we have oyo, which is an alteration of the kata. In these figures, the defender actually places the opponent's left hand down into the defenders right armpit, capturing the opponent's arm and then pushing down.

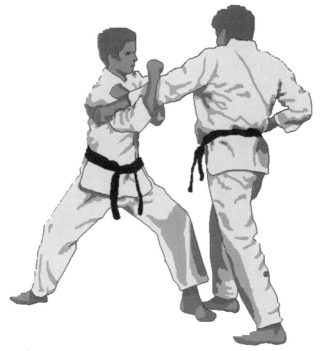

Figure 7 (This is oyo)

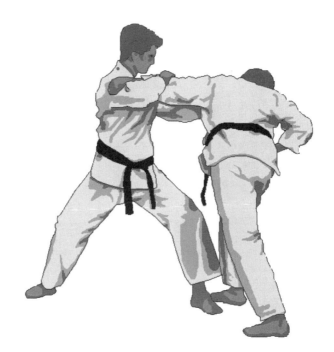

Figure 8

This alteration, used as an example, is not in the traditional performance of this kata. You see no part in the sequence from Kata Figure 6 to Kata Figure 10 where the defender is actually pushing the opponent's hand down into the crevice of his bent elbow, making the hand slide by, as described before, to the side of the defender's head immediately before attacking. The oyo here is that the hand actually opens, and if you will look at Figure 8, he has opened his left hand and he pushes down on the backside of the elbow and strikes the side of the opponent's head. This is oyo. So actually looking at Figures 9, 10, 11, you have oyo, not bunkai.

Oyo emerges when the student analyzes and breaks down a technique seeking the most fluid and efficient way to get in to the technique and explore what develops after that. Oyo is driven by doing what your natural instincts tell you what to do after you have gained complete control of any particular technique.

The best explanation of the concept of oyo is to go to Kata Figure 8 and compare it with Figure 5. This is a block. It is a block whether you do it on the left side or you do it on the right side, it is a block and has always been a block. That's bunkai.

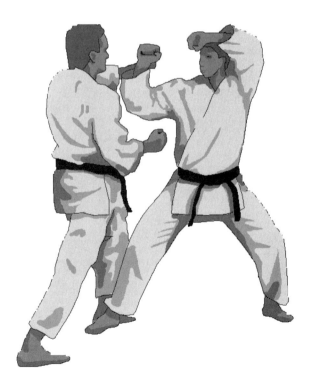

Figure 9

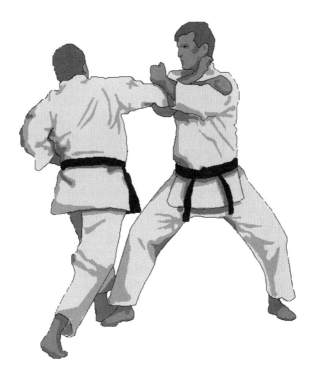

Figure 10

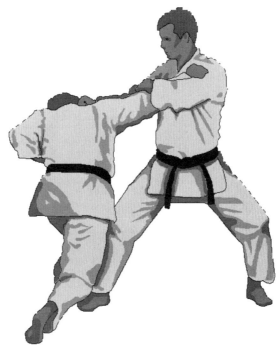

Figure 11

If you look at Figures 12, 13, 14 and 15, these figures are actually the kata done solo as shown in Kata Figures 24, 25 and 26. This is oyo in the old Japanese style. This demonstrates an Okinawa-type wrap-around knife-hand block; this block is executed as a double knife-hand block done in cat stance as shown in Figure 12.

If you accidentally capture the opponent's reverse punch as you wrap around with your forearm, making the stop as shown in Figure 13, you will actually stop and capture the hand. Capturing the opponent's hand is oyo. However, should you just brush the punch to the side simultaneous with your block with the right hand up by the right ear, which would require impeccable timing with the opponent's punching attack, you have bunkai. If you push down with your left hand as shown in Figure 13, a movement that is not in the kata at this point, and execute a strike or block to the side of the attacker's neck, you have oyo.

What Figure 15 actually is would be considered oyo. This oyo has nothing to do with the technique right out of the kata, in a manner of speaking.

It is oyo because it shows in Figure 13 that he does not go down any further than his elbow and then does a spear-hand thrust to the throat. But in Figure 16, the hand down is pushed down below that, which is not in the kata, and this makes it oyo. Most people will say that that is bunkai. No, bunkai would be keeping it in the context of Figure 13. Which he is capable of doing, but the margin of error is much greater.

Kata Figures

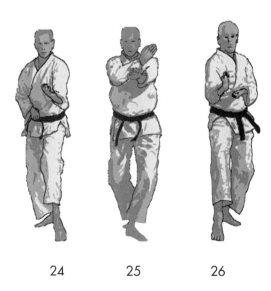

24   25   26

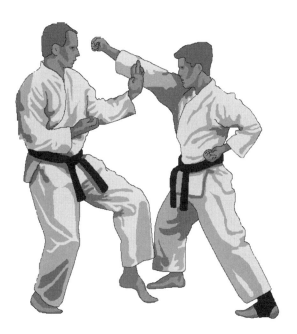

Figure 12

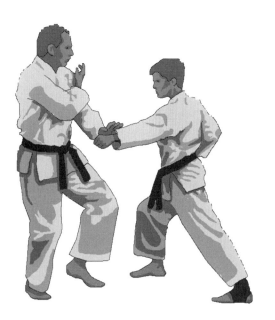

Figure 13 (This is bunkai. Capturing the opponent's hand would make it oyo.)

If an opponent is attacking you, you must be right on the mark. It requires a bull's-eye to be able to do Figure 13. However in Figure 16, the performer can be off center a little bit and still make your spear-hand thrust work.

This is where people have gotten into oyo because bunkai is too technical to make work exactly right in a self-defense or true combat situation. For bunkai to work in combat, the timing has to be exactly perfect, the attack full force, as well as everything else coming together to have a climax right at Kata Figure 15. Most of the time, in real situations, it is not going to work that way.

It could also be that the defender has grabbed the attacker's left hand with his left hand. He then goes to the outside, goes down and comes in with a spear-hand thrust. This is oyo. It could be that the defender just made a technique up from a jujitsu move, such as a rolling of the wrist, pushing down and following with a spear-hand thrust. Now the defender's left hand is going to be just as found in Kata Figure 13.

Oyo is manifested when the student creates something out of kata; this is neither good nor bad, but it's not bunkai. Oyo is indeed a practical part of kata as long as it does not get too bizarre.

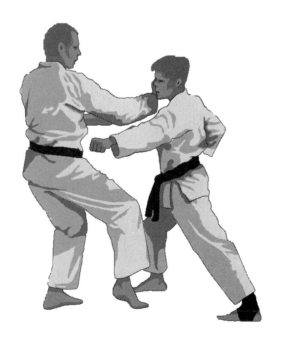

Figure 14

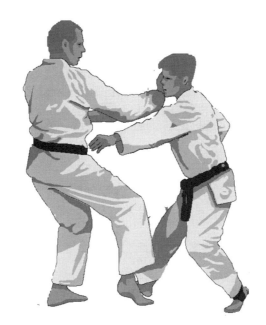

Figure 15

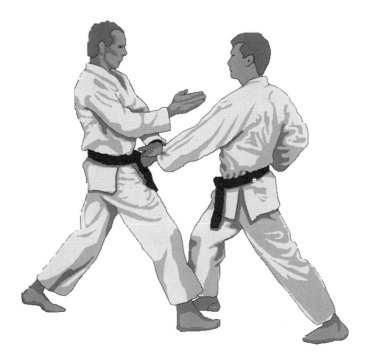

Figure 16

DEMONSTRATING HENKA

Henka is a variation and change in the kata developed from the techniques.

Henka can be a confusing concept. If the kata is changed at all, then oyo would be the various applications of a particular technique. Henka is a variation and change developed from the technique. Henka is not the hidden technique. Henka accounts for the human factor, the human variable. It is the human additive to the kata formula that makes everyone's kata different.

It must be remembered that henka can be anything. Anything that the practitioner makes up is henka. Any variation or self-interpretation of a technique is henka. The henka themselves, amongst a certain population of students doing the same kata, will be different. Henka will vary from student to student just like when we were discussing the earlier example of the seven students with seven different answers. Seven different henkas, definitions and interpretations, and not one of them came up with the actual meaning of bunkai.

Henka is your personal interpretation and this is what most people call bunkai. Henka is the definition of the exceptions made to a kata. More than likely, today, when an instructor teaches a variation of a kata, they are actually most likely teaching the student henka, not a kakushi or even oyo.

If a student of kata were changing or was developing a variation of a technique, this would be considered henka. However, if the student actually stumbled across the hidden part in doing their kata without knowing or realizing it, this could still be considered to be the hidden part.

A sensei is like a conductor of an orchestra. Like the techniques within kata, the conductor wants you to read the notes of the music you are playing while watching his baton. The conductor is certainly not playing the notes for you. The students are the instruments. A symphony conductor does not play the instruments, his job is to listen for the sour notes and identify from where they came.

Like sour notes from an orchestra, henka could be misinterpreted as a derogatory term in certain instances. The point is that henka is just as valid a part of kata as any other part; the conflict is when someone makes up a part and then calls this created part bunkai. While they may be almost correct, or near correct, they are not doing the bunkai. The instructor is merely doing his own thing, his own interpretation of a kata, if it even resembles the original at all. While these variations and changes are developed from the techniques, they are still not the hidden techniques, the kakushi.

DEMONSTRATING KAKUSHI

At the heart of kata, the same movement will have the three different interpretations: oyo, henka and bunkai. In a certain sense, bunkai could even be considered a non-interpretation. Because of the nature of "secret teachings" or "hidden techniques," it is extraordinarily rare that a true teacher will ever reveal the kakushi to a kata. Kakushi is something that is never actually seen, yet it is always there. Most people call it one of the other three elements because they do not really, and will never know of the true hidden part. Kakushi is the missing part of the kata puzzle that so many call bunkai.

The kakushi is never shown in the kata. It is most often something that must be given. Kakushi is the hidden technique within a kata that has always been there but is not seen until someone, likely an old teacher will say, "Let me show you what the hidden technique in this kata is." Once you learn the kakushi, it never varies.

When we observe Figures 17, 18 and 19, we see no variation from the original kata at all. When we consider Figures 20 and 21 and 22 we have kakushi. In this case we have an example a technique of taking somebody down while making a simple turn.

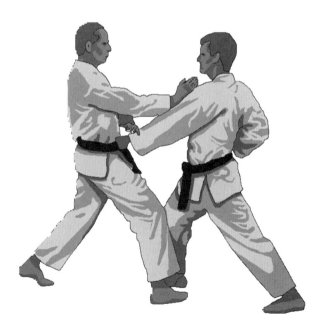

Figure 17

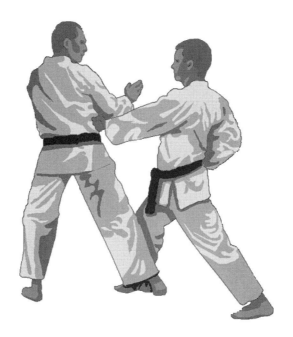

Figure 18

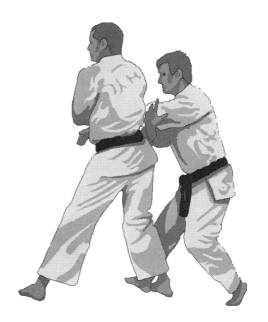

Figure 19

Often when we attempt to explain the kakushi of this particular move, we cannot. For the simple reason that there is none. Here is where many people would just make up a "hidden technique" which in this particular kata is often to come to the outside of the hand, grab a hold, pushing down and do the spear-hand thrust. This is hogwash.

What the kata practitioner has done here is considered to be henka. This is also one of the few techniques in this particular kata that would be considered to have a kakushi part to it—however, we will cover this in a moment.

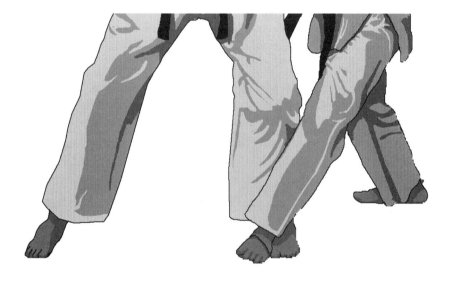

Figure 20 (This is kukushi)

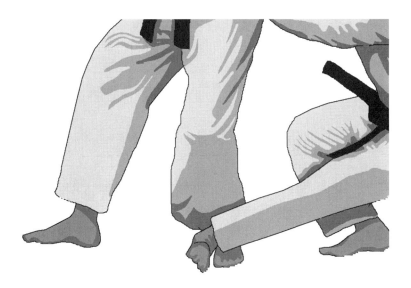

Figure 21 (This is kukushi)

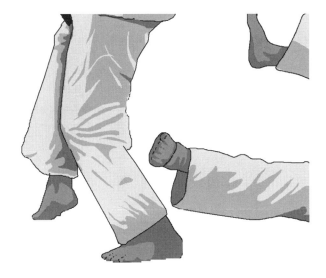

Figure 22 (Kukushi completed)

The bunkai can be observed in Figures 23, 24, and 25. Oyo comes into view in Figure 26, because the defender changes his hands from the original position of the kata when he turns around. You can see this in Figure 27.

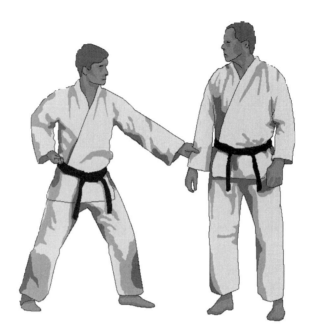

Figure 23

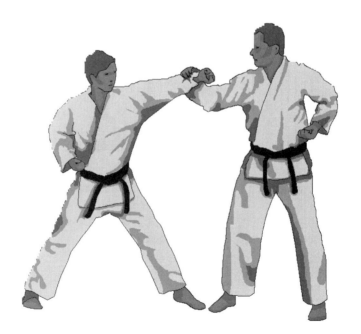

Figure 24

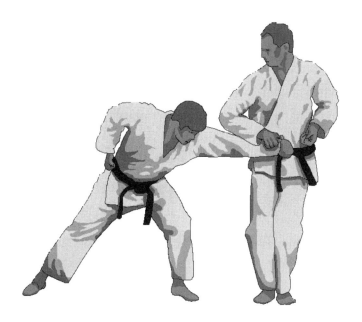

Figure 25

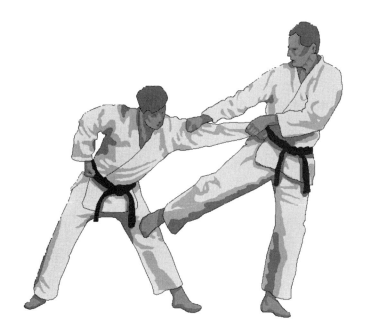

Figure 26

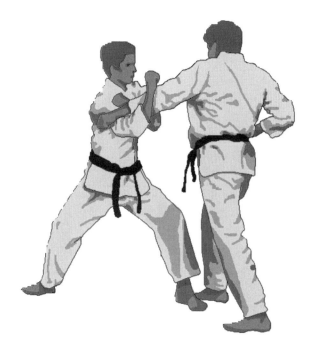

Figure 27

If we get into the hidden technique, the kakushi, it would be lifting the hand up as it is coming in and executing an elbow strike. Many people that do this particular kata say that at this point, Figure 29, another attacker is coming from the front and so once the leg technique is complete you have dispatched him. Now you turn 180 degrees and you block the next attacker. We have heard this, "you block the next attacker" so many times. Unfortunately, most students will buy this (or rather pay for it!). What has really been missed and unnoticed is the hidden technique that they have not seen. Only someone who knows, perhaps a master, can show the student the hidden technique of the finishing as seen in Figure 29.

Often brighter students, who may likely not be too familiar with the kata, will ask a sensei if the henka is when another opponent is coming. It is not uncommon for a student to ask, "Sensei, after you have done this sequence, what is to be done here?" Most students will then ask the teacher, "I am blocking another attacker, right?" Unfortunately at this point, most teachers will say, "yes." Some know better, some know not. Some care not to know at all and some know and will never say.

If there is a hidden move, it would be hidden within the motions of Figures 28 and 29.

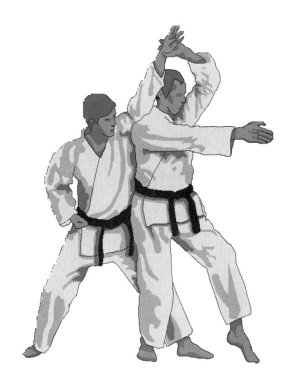

Figure 28

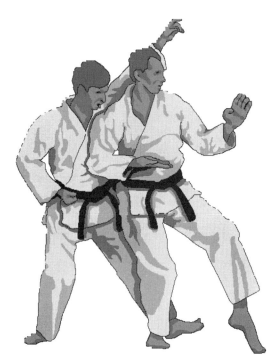

Figure 29

There may be a kakushi in the take-down demonstrated in Figures 30, 31, and 32.

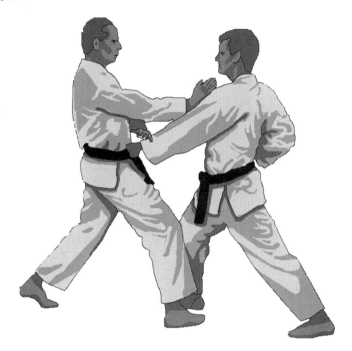

Figure 30

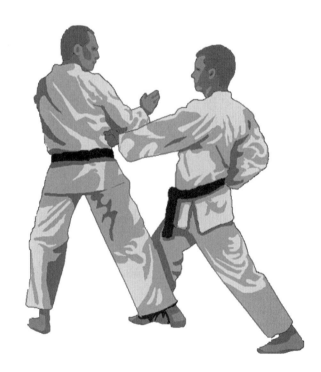

Figure 31

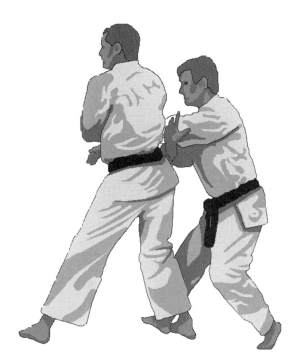

Figure 32

There can be an elbow strike executed in Figure 33. Here taking the opponent down and hitting him, as in seen in Figure 34. To add some further depth to this, there may also be the same hidden technique on the turn around.

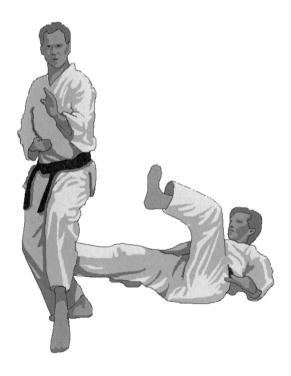

Figure 33

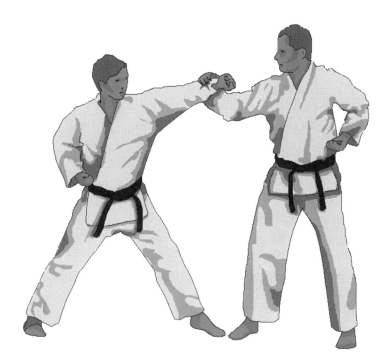

Figure 34

CONCLUSION: THE PRACTICAL APPLICATION OF BUNKAI

In battle it matters not whether you are doing oyo, kakushi or bunkai. The successful application of the technique is obviously the only thing that really matters.

So many people today have changed the aged techniques originally meant to be communicated through the form of kata. They have been changed to fit into the future. They are calling it bunkai, but this is not bunkai.

Unless a teacher has made up their own entire kata and placed within that kata their own proven and practical techniques, and then continue to teach it precisely from decade to decade, you do not have bunkai. At their core, most kata today are vestiges of battle-proven techniques from a time when weapons influenced the proximity of combat. Today this is commonly referred to as Close Quarters Combat (CQB).

The martial masters of old knew in great detail the efficacy of technique—what worked and what did not. They then took this practical knowledge and buried them in their kata, anticipating that the wisdom gained from their experience would survive for generations. However, in modern times, how often does a person incur aggressors "on the street" and get to practice making a technique work? Battlefield experiences today are for the most part left only to Navy SEALs, bodyguards, brawlers and rebels.

Kata, and most martial arts fundamentals are based on self-defense moves that have been proven in combat over hundreds, in some cases thousands, of years. Some of these moves, which were repeatedly proved successful back then, may not apply in today's society at all. A kakushi designed to defend against a sword is irrelevant today—no one fights with swords anymore.

People have changed and modified most kata to fit into today's society. When this happens, you no longer have bunkai. If a kata is altered in any way, then it cannot be bunkai. If my pants are altered to fit you, then they are not my pants anymore. Bunkai is when I can get into my pants no matter who has worn them, as long as they have not been altered. We may have two pairs of pants exactly alike. The bunkai was cutting them exactly alike from the same pattern, perhaps in two different sizes, but as soon as they are altered, you have henka.

One of the concepts we should briefly take time to clarify is that there is no superiority or inferiority between bunkai and oyo. Should a student have the time and discipline to commit years of study and practice to kata, they will find that the bunkai is taught so that they can eventually learn the kakushi. The teacher teaches the oyo so they can survive. Again, keep in mind that one cannot have the correct oyo without the bunkai.

We were writing earlier about proven battlefield techniques. Today's battlefields, for the most part, are populated with police officers.

Craig Sensei discussed the practical application of kata, in the light of his 16 years of experience teaching self-defense for a large metropolitan police department as well as the federal government for nine years after that. He said that; "When I first started teaching young police officers, I had all of these great ideas about how to teach them valuable self-defense skills because I knew the "bunkai" from my particular martial discipline. It was not too long before street officers would come back and say that the techniques I taught, the oyo which were derived from the bunkai I knew, did not exactly always work on the street."

Craig Sensei continued that the instructor in me knew that these techniques should work, that they have to work. And yet, consistently these professionals would say that, "No, I am sorry, but I got beaten the other night and what you taught me did not work in this particular circumstance." As time went by, it became imperative that the techniques, the bunkai, be modified for the safety of the officers for whom the sensei was responsible. Once a modification, any modification occurred, there was no longer bunkai; now we had oyo.

Speaking more about his experience teaching police officers, Craig Sensei explained that when he broke away from the bunkai and began exploring the oyo, everything started working on the street for these officers. When we began to modify techniques in consideration of the realities an officer faces when his survival instincts have taken over, real world factors such as the entry, the off-balance and the timing become a necessary the part of the technique in order to allow a suspect to be taken into custody safely and with minimum force.

Perhaps we should look to *iaido*, the way of the sword or even more specifically *iaijujitsu*, the practical use of the sword, to further this point. In today's society obviously, the sword as a weapon is largely a dinosaur. No one runs around anymore carrying swords, much less big knives. They may do it on TV and in the movies, and there may certainly be a few crazy and insane people running around our cities secretly wanting to be ninjas and pretending to be the Highlander, but for the most part the practical application of sword fighting is useless (however, the character and spiritual development from practicing with the sword can be enormous, ask any kendoist).

These swordsmen, practiced or not, often imagine all of the various draws, parries and strikes of their sword. The fact is that what they are imagining or practicing relates in no way to any part of our society today as we know it. In many cases, sword bunkai survives within very old styles such as Mu gai ryu, because it is being successfully perpetuated and learned exactly as it was taught with out variation. In contrast, The All Japan Kendo Federation has changed their kata so often, within the last generation alone, to adopt to the contemporary demands of modern times—the position of the hands, the position of the feet, the position of the sword, they have all been changed and there is no bunkai anymore, there is just oyo and henka.

The reader should be leery of assuming that what we are attempting to communicate through this book is that what is being discussed here is absolutely correct and that instruction to the contrary is absolutely wrong. As with all things, this is not so black and white. We do however think that it is fair, from experience and research both, that tough questions must be asked. Do the majority of martial arts students truly know what they are doing? How can this be the case if there is such as vast population of people out there, students and scholars alike, that do not understand the intended differences in the ideas represented in the words, bunkai, oyo, henka and kakushi.

It is important to the authors to communicate to the reader that the act of doing oyo or henka is no less relevant than bunkai, or even kakushi. However, do not call it bunkai unless you are doing it exactly as you learned the kata. It is with some 99.9 percent certainty that most kata's performed today are done oblivious to the core practical application or intention—the kakushi. And virtually every vague attempt to execute kakushi is inappropriately referred to as the bunkai.

CHAPTER SIX

Waza Descriptions

In previous books, the attacker was referred to as *uohidaohi* or *uke* and the defender as *shidachi* or *tori*. In our research, we did not find a suitable Okinawan term for attacker and defender. To keep from confusing the issue, we simply refer to the attacker as the attacker and the defender as the defender. Be aware that not all bunkai movements correspond exactly with the kata movements.

In dissecting the first waza from the kata (which is shown in its entirety at the back of this book), Figures 17 and 18 demonstrate the movements on the right side. Although the left side is not performed in the kata, the bunkai is equally effective from both sides. In most katas, the waza is performed on the right side. (NOTE: The dominance of the right hand was driven by cultural demands.)

WAZA 1

Figures 35–40 corresponds with Kata Figures 17–24 from the complete kata sequence. The action begins with the attacker reaching for the defender's right wrist with his left hand, preparatory to striking with his right hand. Figure 36 shows the defender stepping back with his left foot to his left while simultaneously raising his right hand to capture the attacker's left wrist between his thumb and index finger. Figure 37 shows the defender bringing his right foot up to his left foot, rotating the attacker's wrist counterclockwise and pulling the attacker off balance to his awaiting left hand. The attacker's hand is now palm up in the defender's left hand. The defender's elbow rests across the attacker's elbow. Kata Figure 21 corresponds with Figure 38. The defender pushes down with his right elbow, continuing to force the attacker off balance. The defender keeps a tight grip with his left hand while sliding his right hand up to just above the attacker's elbow. He then lifts the attacker's left arm while simultaneously lifting his right foot to deliver a side stomp kick to just above the attacker's left knee. Kata Figures 23 and 24 correspond with Figures 39 and 40. The defender now steps to the center of the attacker's body with his right foot while continuing to lift the attacker's left arm and simultaneously turns his body 90 degrees to his left (see Figure 39). He then releases the attacker's left hand, lowers into a cat stance and delivers a right elbow strike to the rear into the attacker's solar plexus (see Figure 40). (NOTE: When performing the elbow strike, the sinking motion of the defender's hips into a proper cat stance automatically forces the attacker off balance.)

Kata Figures

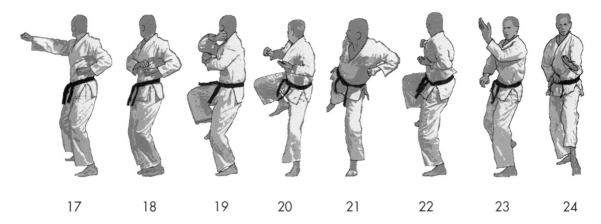

| 17 | 18 | 19 | 20 | 21 | 22 | 23 | 24 |

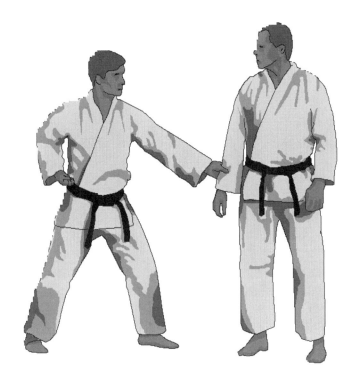

Figure 35

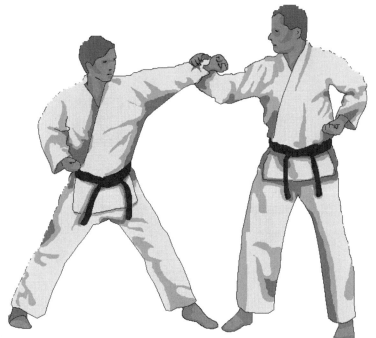

Figure 36

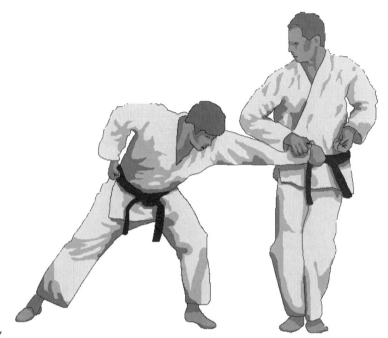

Figure 37

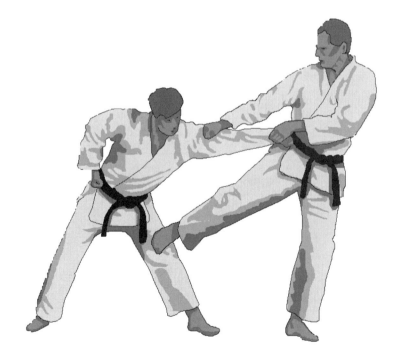

Figure 38

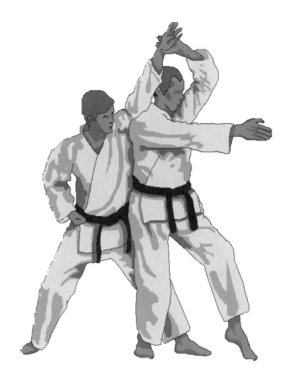

Figure 39

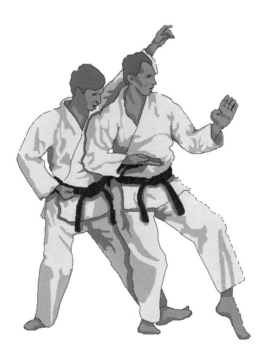

Figure 40

WAZA 2

This waza corresponds with Kata Figures 6–10 in the kata sequence (Kata Figures 6–10 are the left side and Kata Figures 11–15 are the right side of the kata sequence). We describe the left side only. The attacker stands in a left forward stance (see Figure 41). In Figure 42, the attacker steps forward with his right foot and strikes at the defender's face with his right fist. Kata Figures 6–8 show the defender stepping forward with his left foot into a left back stance, performing a U-block and blocking the attacker's right forearm with his left forearm (see Figure 42 again). The attacker now delivers a left-hand punch to the defender's face (see Figure 43). The defender uses his left hand to perform an outside-inside block across his body, stopping at the attacker's wrist (see Kata Figure 9) while shifting from a back stance to a modified forward stance. This movement is performed by rotating on the ball of the right foot with the left foot remaining in its original position.

Kata Figures

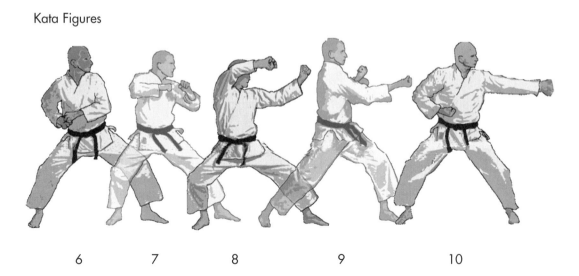

| 6 | 7 | 8 | 9 | 10 |

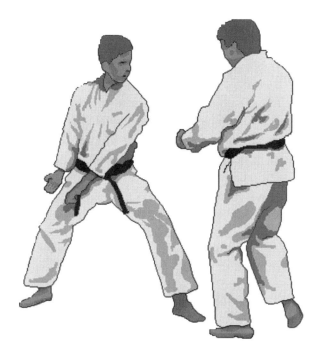

Figure 41

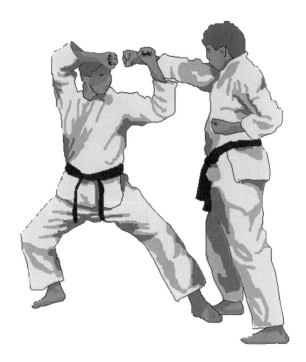

Figure 42

In Figure 44, the defender does an outside-inside block with his right forearm striking the attacker's left elbow with the bottom of his right fist. At the same time, he uses his left hand to place the attacker's wrist into the bend of his right elbow. He now pushes down on the attacker's elbow with his right fist while simultaneously shifting back to the original back stance. (NOTE: The shift keeps the attacker off balance). He then secures the attacker's wrist into the fold of his right arm by pushing with his left hand to his right and pulling with his right hand into his chest. This action secures the attacker's bent wrist tightly against his right breast (see Kata Figure 10 and Figure 45). Next, the defender shifts into a horse stance while maintaining a firm grip on the attacker's wrist, and delivers a left-hand punch (with the first two knuckles of his fist) half an inch below the attacker's left ear (that is, where the carotid artery is located). (NOTE: An option may exist where the defender delivers a back fist strike to the attacker's left temple. Craig Sensei was originally taught this particular waza as a punch, not a back-fist strike.) Figures 46–48 demonstrate the waza from the right side.

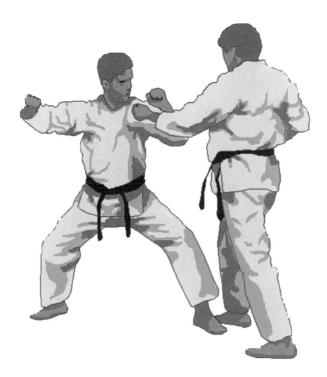

Figure 43

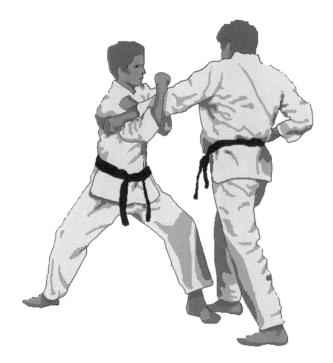

Figure 44

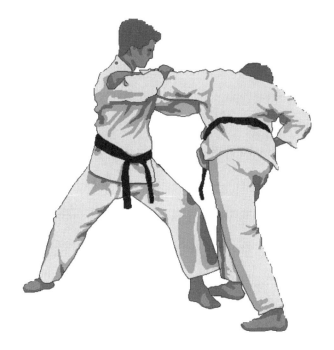

Figure 45

Waza 2 (from the Right Hand Side)

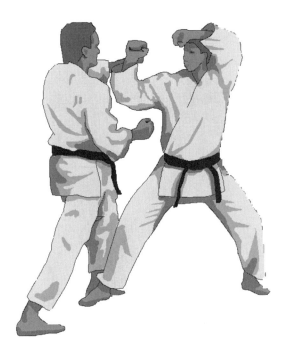

Figure 46

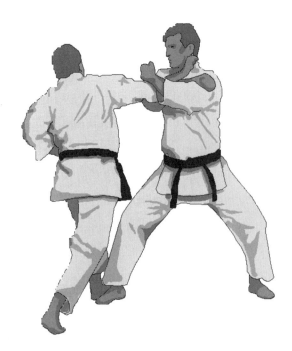

Figure 47

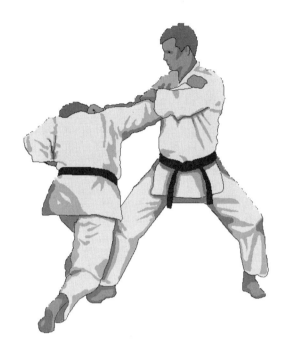

Figure 48

Kata Figures

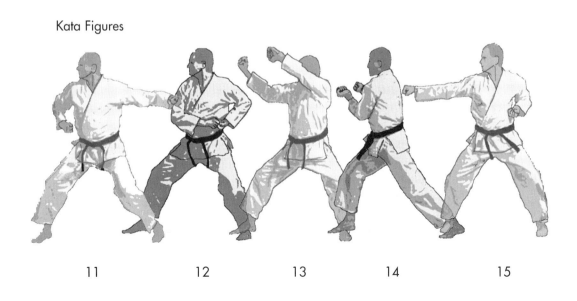

11   12   13   14   15

WAZA 3

This waza corresponds with Kata Figures 24–26 in the kata sequence. In Figure 49, the attacker steps forward with his right foot and delivers a punch with his right hand to the defender's face. (NOTE: This motion can also be done without stepping forward.) The defender immediately steps forward into a left cat stance and blocks the attack with a left knife-hand strike. The defender's right hand is now palm up and on level with his solar plexus with the fingers pointing toward the attacker. The attacker now delivers a left-hand punch to the defender's solar plexus. The defender uses the palm of his left hand to block this attack. The defender raises his right hand above his left shoulder, thereby allowing his right elbow to protect his solar plexus (see Figure 50).

Kata Figures

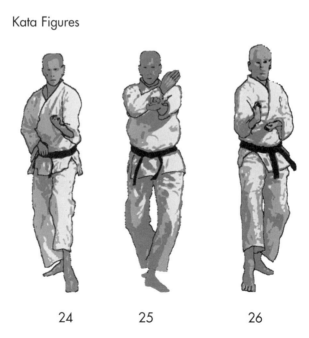

24   25   26

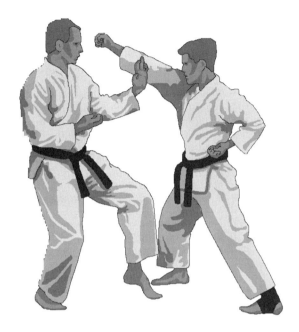

Figure 49

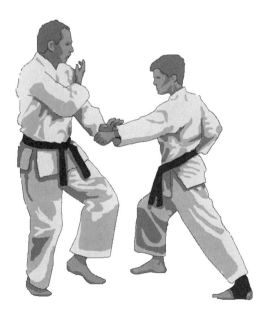

Figure 50

These motions are all done while maintaining the original left cat stance. The defender now steps forward with his right foot into a right cat stance and delivers a knife-hand strike to the right side of the attacker's neck one half inch below the ear on the carotid artery (see Figures 51 and 52). The defender's left hand is now palm up on level with his solar plexus with the fingers pointing toward the attacker. Kata Figures 27–30 represent the same movement from the left side.

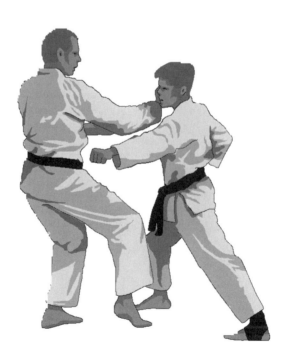

Figure 57

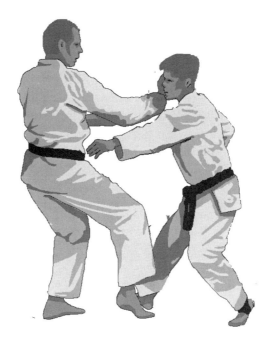

Figure 52

WAZA 4

This waza corresponds with Kata Figures 30–36 in the kata sequence. Starting with Figure 53, the attacker steps forward with his right foot and punches to the defender's face with his right hand. (NOTE: The attacker does not need to step forward to make the technique work.) The defender steps forward into a left cat stance and blocks with his left hand as in the previous bunkai. The attacker now punches at the defender's chest with his left hand. The defender uses a pushing-down block with the palm of his left hand as he steps forward with his right foot (see Figure 54). (Although it is not shown in the drawings, the defender places his fingers in the attacker's palm hand and his thumb on top of the attacker's index finger knuckle.)

Kata Figures

"Kiai"

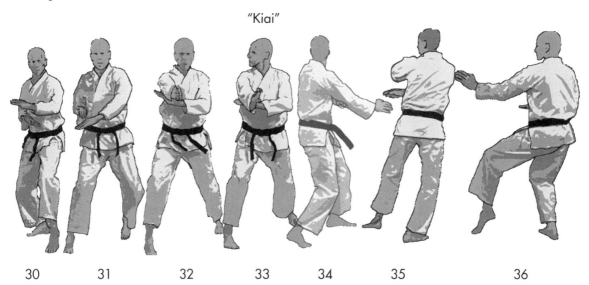

| 30 | 31 | 32 | 33 | 34 | 35 | 36 |

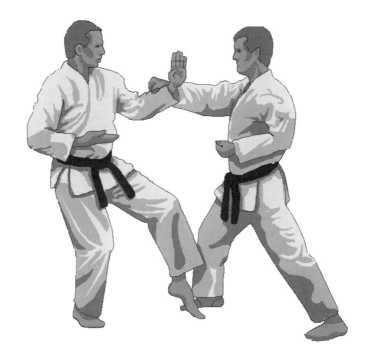

Figure 53

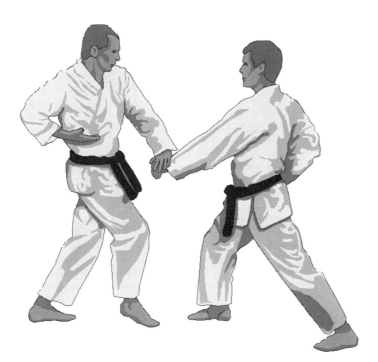

Figure 54

The defender twists the attacker's hand counterclockwise while simultaneously delivering a right spear-hand thrust to his throat (see Figures 55 and 56). Kata Figures 29–32 show the actual kata movements. (NOTE: For the next bunkai series, the attacker must step through with his right foot.) The defender then pushes down with his right elbow to the top of the attacker's right elbow, thereby breaking his balance. The defender releases the attacker's left wrist and places his right foot behind the attacker's right heel at a 90-degree angle (see Figure 57). The defender pivots 270 degrees counterclockwise into a left cat stance with a double knife-hand block (see Kata Figures 34–36).

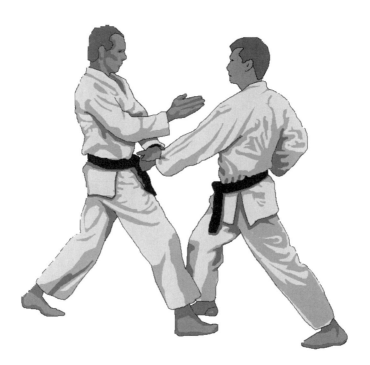

Figure 55

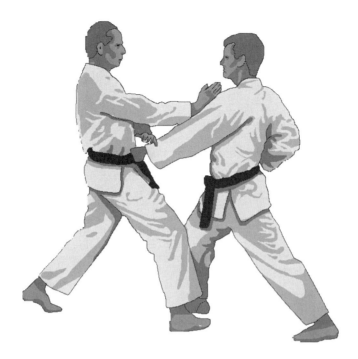

Figure 56

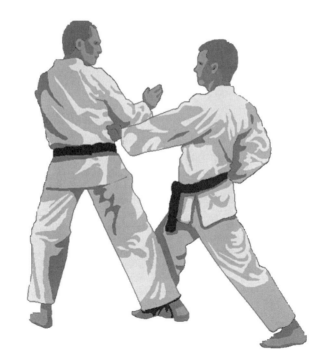

Figure 57

Figures 59 and 60 are accomplished after he steps behind the attacker's right (advanced) foot. The defender simply bends his knee, the sinking motion of his hips into a proper cat stance automatically forces the attacker off balance.

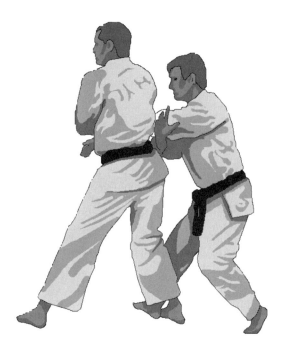

Figure 58

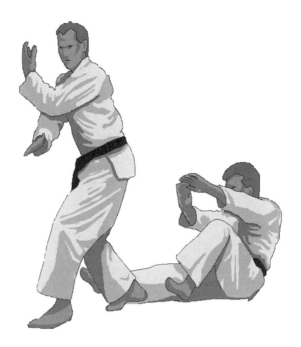

Figure 59

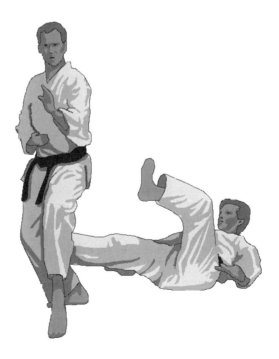

Figure 60

Figures 61–63 represents the defender's footwork if the attacker has not stepped through with his right foot but rather has his left foot forward. The defender simply steps forward with his left foot instead of his right and delivers a right spear-hand thrust to the attacker's throat. The defender now places his left foot behind the attacker's left heel (Figure 61). The defender makes a 180-degree turn clockwise into a right cat stance with a double knife-hand block (Figures 62 and 63). The defender may also strike to the rear with his left elbow to the attacker's solar plexus or face as he falls. This elbow technique can be executed from the right side, but the timing is much more complex and requires advanced practice.

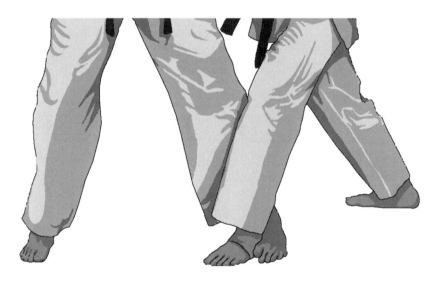

Figure 61

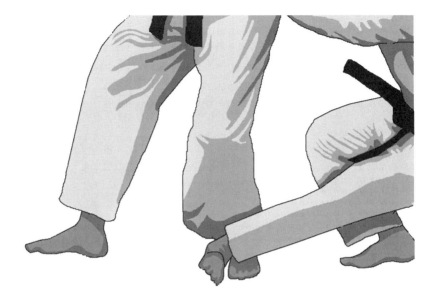

Figure 62

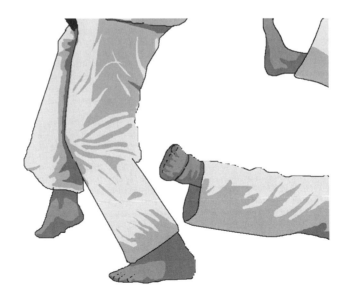

Figure 63

WAZAS 5 AND 6

These two wazas correspond to Kata Figures 38–44 in the kata sequence. These two wazas in the kata are nothing more than waza 3 performed on the left side by moving into left cat stance, stepping forward at a 45-degree angle and striking the right side of the attacker's neck. The defender then steps back, turns 135 degrees into a right cat stance and double knife-hand blocks. He then steps 45 degrees with his left foot into a left cat stance and strikes the left side of the attacker's neck.

Kata Figures

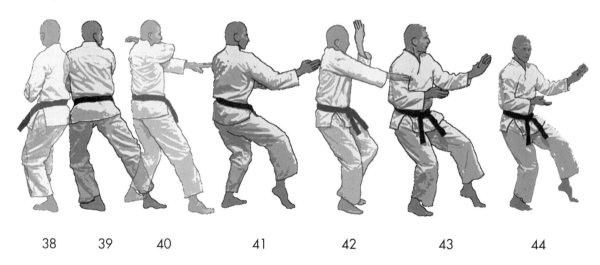

38   39   40   41   42   43   44

WAZA 7

This waza begins with the attacker standing behind the defender. He seizes the defender's right shoulder with his left hand and starts to pull, thereby turning the defender's body clockwise. As the defender turns his head, he sees that the attacker intends to strike with his right hand (see Figure 64). In Figure 65, the defender steps back with his right foot and raises his right hand to the attacker's chin.

Kata Figures

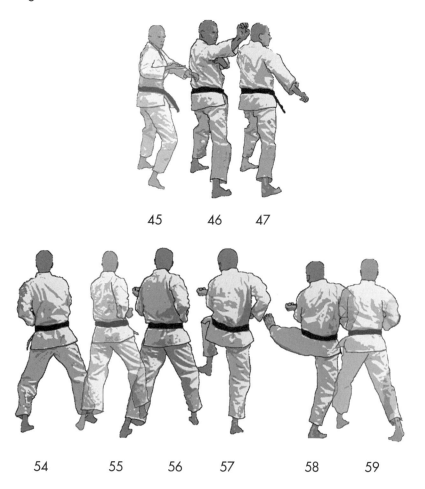

45   46   47

54   55   56   57   58   59

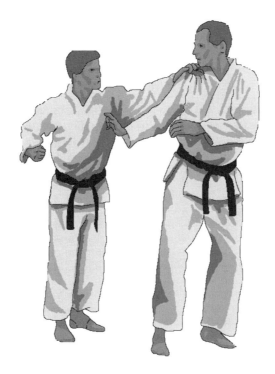

Figure 64

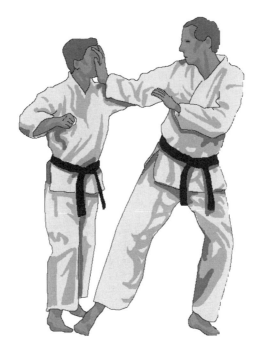

Figure 65

In Figure 66, the attacker has completed his punch. The defender, however, has pushed the attacker's chin while blocking the punch with his left hand. In Figure 67, the defender grasps the attacker's right wrist turning it slightly clockwise so that the outside of his elbow is pulled tightly into the defender's right breast thereby creating an arm-bar (NOTE: This motion is very important in that it forces the attacker off balance to the defender's front right diagonal area.) The defender reaches outside and behind the attacker's right knee (see Figure 68).

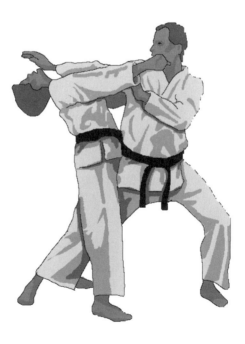

Figure 66

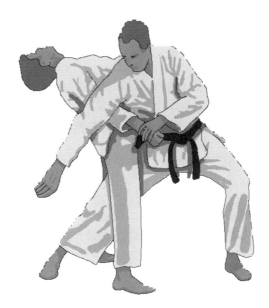

Figure 67

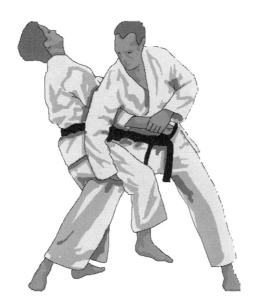

Figure 68

In Figure 69, the defender completes his movement behind the attacker's right knee by sliding his fist behind the knee and lifting upward with his forearm in a scooping motion. (NOTE: The defender does not grab the knee.) The defender continues pulling while shifting his hips to his left, forcing the attacker over his right leg (see Figure 69). Figure 70 shows the completion of the movement shown in Kata Figure 48. Even though Figure 71 appears to be placing the attacker in front of the defender, it is important to note that the defender releases the attacker when he reaches the front right diagonal area. Figure 72 shows the completion of the waza with a kick to the attacker's groin using the ball of the right foot. (NOTE: The kick must be between the attacker's legs thereby catching the scrotum, and not to the top of the pelvic bone.

Kata Figures 54–59 show this waza on the left side omitting the initial attack as shown in Kata Figures 45-47 on the right side.

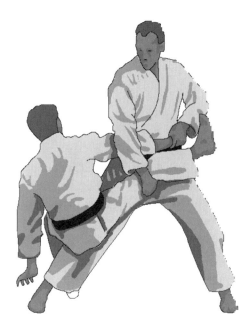

Figure 69

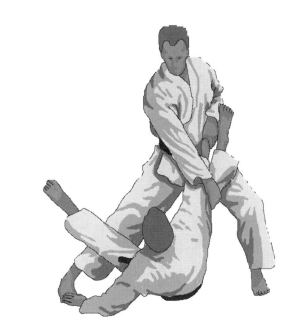

Figure 70

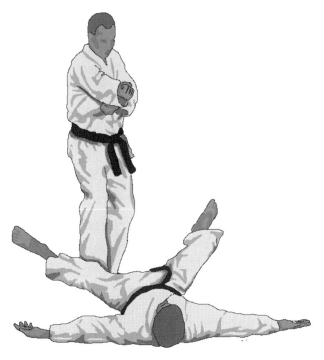

Figure 71

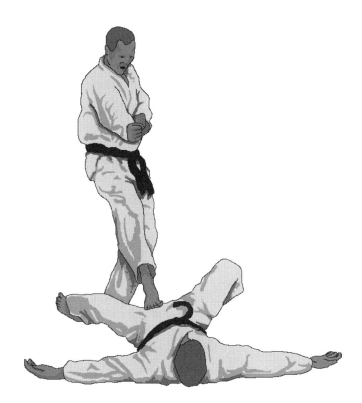

Figure 72

WAZA 8

This waza corresponds to Kata Figures 60–65 in the kata sequence. In Figure 73 the attacker grabs the defender's right bicep with his right hand. The defender steps back with his left foot while performing a modified augmented forearm block with his right arm. In this modification, the defender secures the attacker's hand with the bottom of his left fist, thus preventing the attacker from releasing his hold on the biceps. This motion, in most cases, forces the attacker to step forward with his right foot to try to regain his balance. Figures 74 and 75 show the completion of the waza when the defender begins his 270-degree turn to his left. This turn causes the attacker to fall to the defender's rear. (Notice that the footwork is the same as Waza 4, see Figures 57 and 58).

Kata Figures

"Kiai"

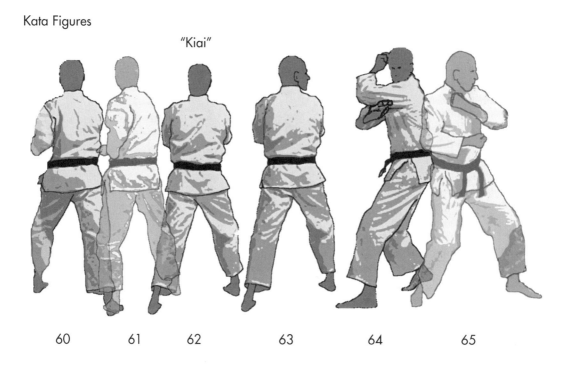

60   61   62   63   64   65

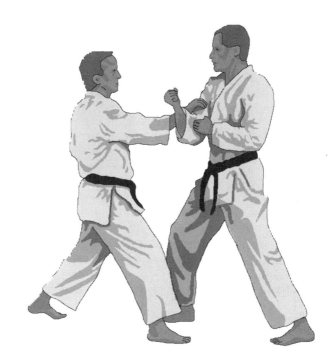

Figure 73

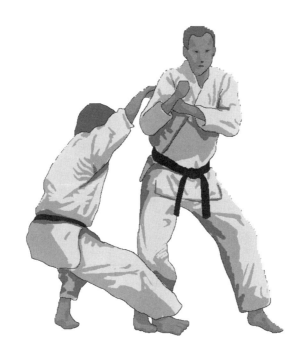

Figure 74

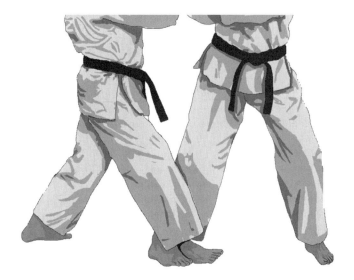

Figure 75

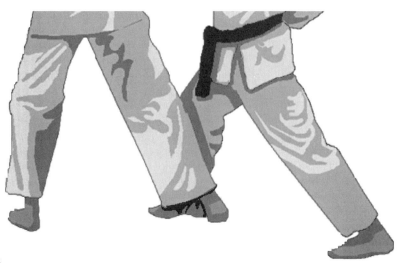

Figure 76

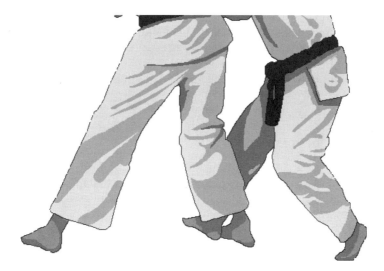

Figure 77

WAZA 9

This waza corresponds to Kata Figures 66–73 in the kata sequence. In Figure 78, the attacker grabs the defender's left wrist with his left hand. In Figures 79 and 80, the defender steps back slightly with his right foot while simultaneously bringing his left hand to his left side, which forces the attacker off balance. As the attacker pulls back, trying regain his balance, the defender raises his left hand in a high blocking motion and seizes the outside of the attacker's left wrist (Figures 81and 82).

Kata Figures

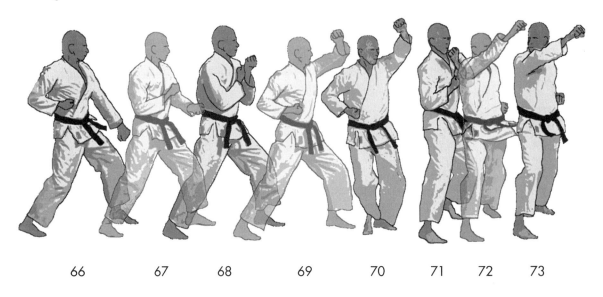

66   67   68   69   70   71   72   73

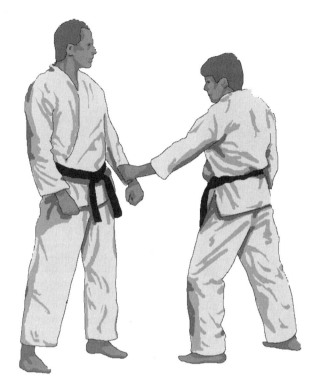

Figure 78

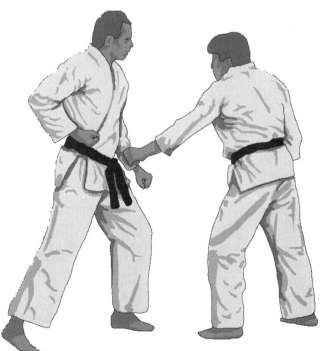

Figure 79

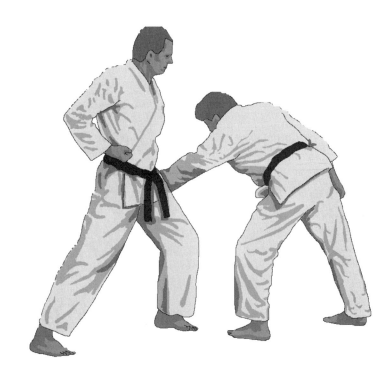

Figure 80

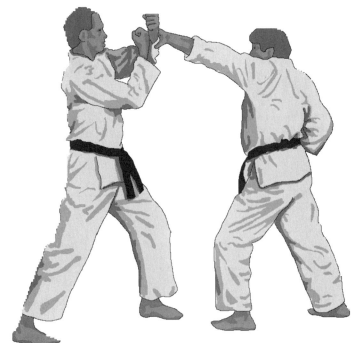

Figure 81

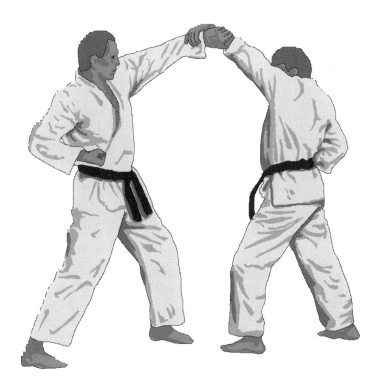

Figure 82

Figures 83, 84, and 85 show a close-up of opening the defender's left hand and seizing the attacker's wrist (see also Kata Figures 69 and 70).

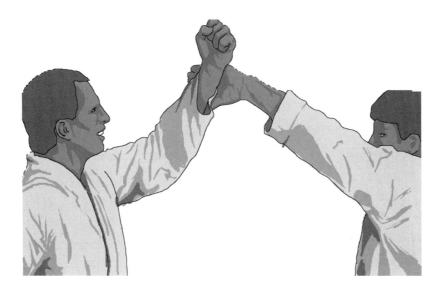

Figure 83

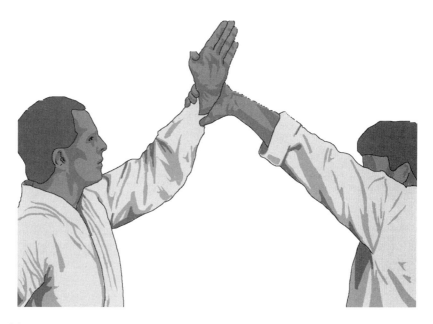

Figure 84

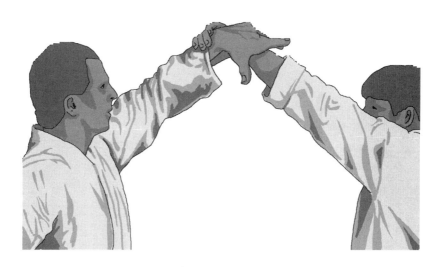

Figure 85

Figures 86and 87show the finishing motion to the waza. After taking a firm grip with his left hand, the defender rotates the attacker's wrist slightly clockwise, steps forward with his right foot and strikes the attacker at his elbow. In the kata, this waza resembles nothing as much as a left down block, left high block, opening and closing of the left high-blocking hand, and stepping through and high blocking with the right hand.

Kata Figures 74–80 show the left side of this waza. Kata Figures 81–82 shows the preparation for the closing bow.

Kata Figures

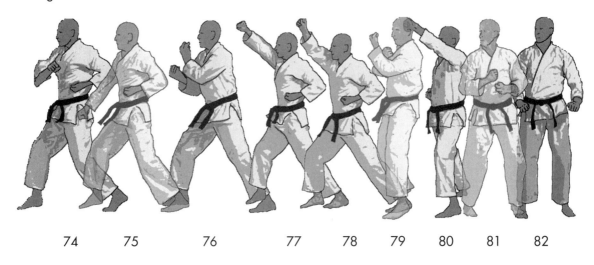

| 74 | 75 | 76 | 77 | 78 | 79 | 80 | 81 | 82 |

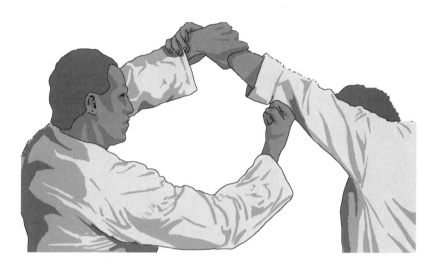

Figure 86

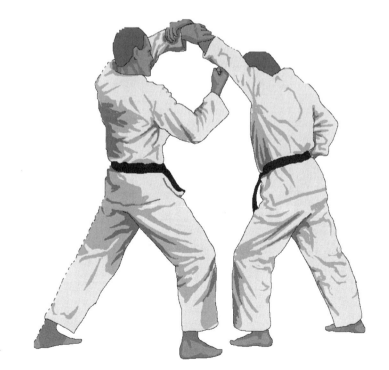

Figure 87

BONUS WAZAS

WAZA 1A

Figures 89–91 are the same as Waza 1 (Figures 35–37) except that the defender does not bring his feet together. In Figure 93, the defender moves his left foot to the left into a modified horse stance. In Figure 95 and 97, the defender continues pulling with his right hand to his left hand, turning the attacker's wrist slightly counterclockwise. The attacker's elbow should be pointing upward; the defender's elbow should be resting on top of the attacker's elbow (see Figure 97 again). In Figure 97, the defender has created a straight arm-bar on his attacker. The defender now presses downward with his elbow until submission (see Figure 98). (NOTE: It is important to maintain correct posture. Do not apply pressure by leaning forward or sideways. Correct pressure is applied by sinking the hips and by lowering the controlling elbow.)

Kata Figures

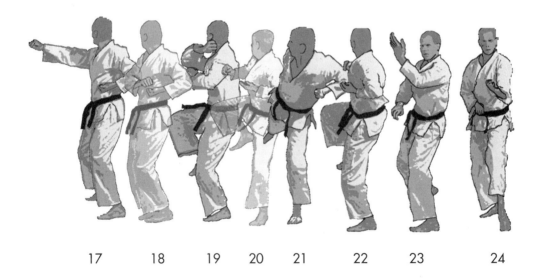

17   18   19   20   21   22   23   24

140

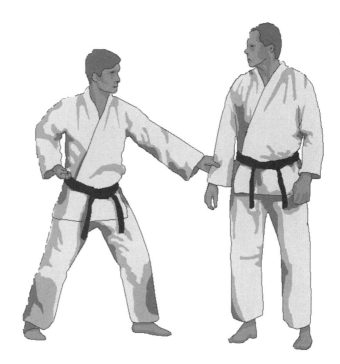

Figure 88 (Same as Figure 35 from Waza 1)

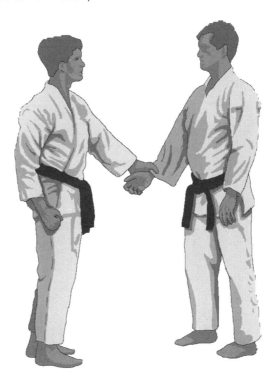

Figure 89

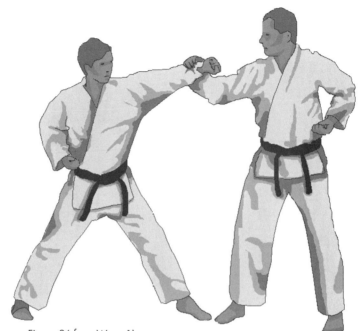

Figure 90 (Same as Figure 36 from Waza 1)

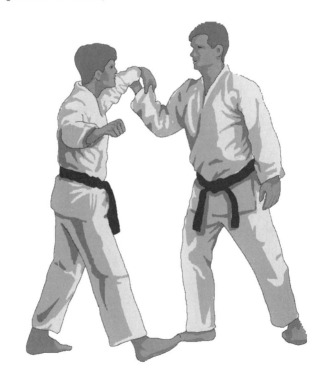

Figure 91

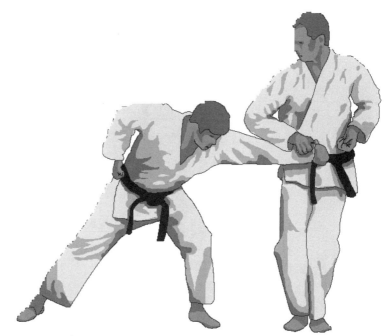

Figure 92 (Same as Figure 37 from Waza 1)

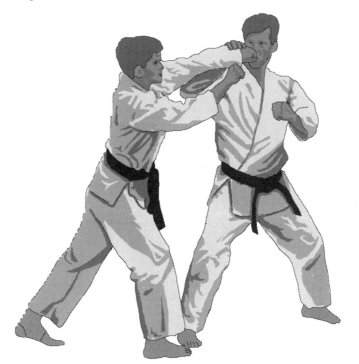

Figure 93

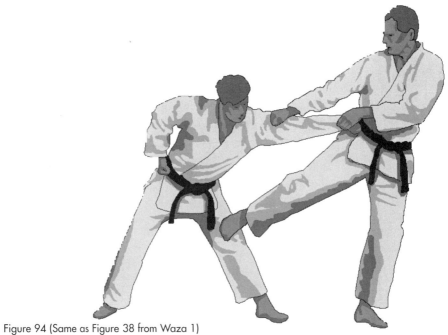

Figure 94 (Same as Figure 38 from Waza 1)

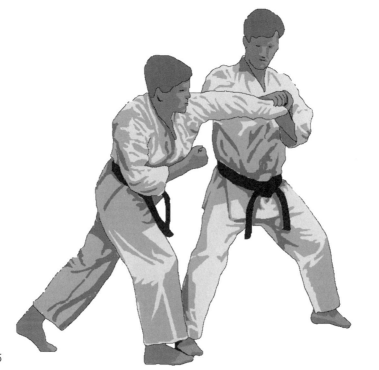

Figure 95

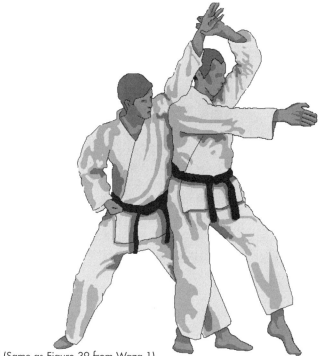

Figure 96 (Same as Figure 39 from Waza 1)

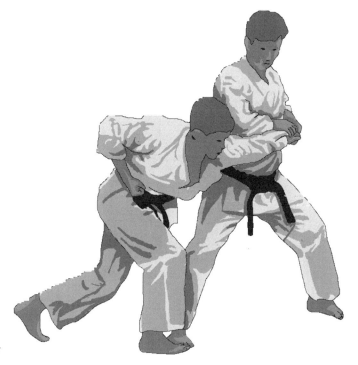

Figure 97

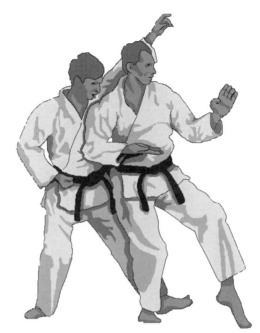

Figure 98 (Same as Figure 40 from Waza 1)

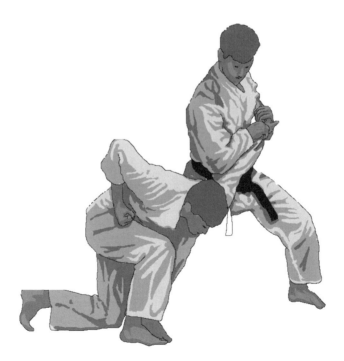

Figure 99

WAZA 8A

Figures 101 and 102 show what is simply another application of Waza 8. After the attacker has grabbed and the defender has performed the augmented block, the attacker releases his grip (see Figure 101). As the defender feels the grip loosening, he pushes immediately down on the attacker's upper forearm. He then slides forward with his right foot and attacks with an augmented back-fist strike to the right side of the attacker's neck (see Figure 103).

Kata Figures

"Kiai"

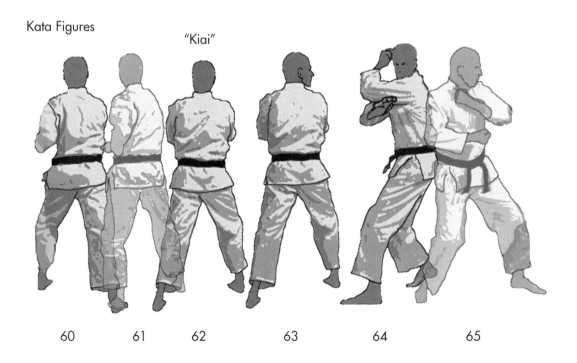

| 60 | 61 | 62 | 63 | 64 | 65 |

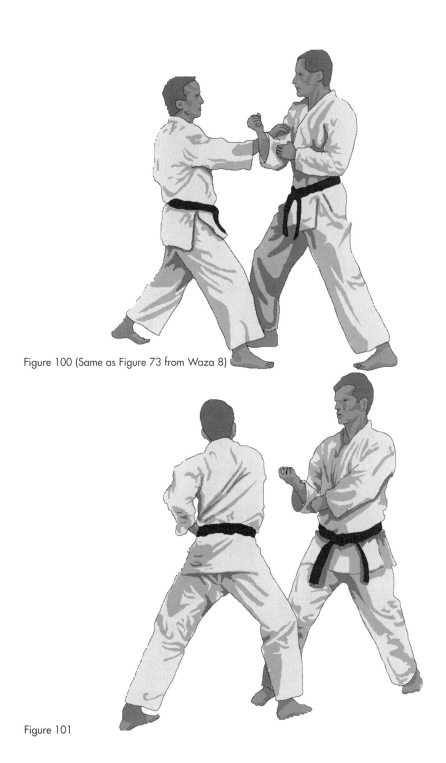

Figure 100 (Same as Figure 73 from Waza 8)

Figure 101

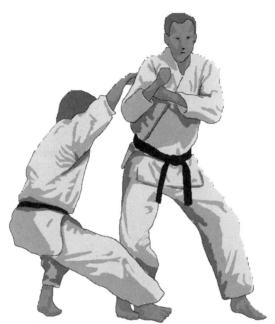

Figure 102 (Same as Figure 74 from Waza 8)

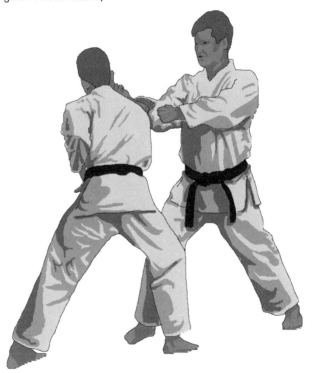

Figure 103

EXPLANATION OF KATA MOVES 1–82

In performing this or any other kata, it is essential that the practitioner turn his head in the direction of his next move, *before* initiating that move. This turning movement assures that his head, and thus his hands, are properly aligned for executing the technique. While the head determines the direction of the hands, the hips determine the direction of the feet.

Figures 1–5 (on p. 154) represent the bow. Figures 6–8 show turning your head to the left, stepping with your left foot to your left into a left back stance, stacking your hands with palms facing each other on your right side and bringing your hands into a U-block. Perform an outside-inside block with your left hand, bringing it to your right shoulder (see Figure 9) while simultaneously performing an outside-inside block with your right hand stopping in the center of your face. Shifting into a *kubadachi* strike with a left straight punch (Figure 10). See Figures 6–10 under Waza 2. The right hand then goes to the right hip. Figures 11 and 12 show turning your head to the right and stacking your hands on your left side. Figures 13–15 are a repeat of Figures 8–10. Figures 16–18 show stepping with your left foot to the center, bringing your feet together and stacking your hands on your left side. Bring your right foot up, side snap kick or side stomp kick with your right foot to your right while simultaneously back fist striking with your right hand (Figures 19–22). Rechamber your right leg to the outside of your right knee. Figure 23 and 24 shows stepping back to your original starting position with your right foot turning counterclockwise 90 degrees to your left into a left cat stance with a left double knife-hand block.

Figures 25–29 shows stepping directly forward into a right cat stance and right double knife hand block, and then stepping directly forward into a left cat stance and a left double knife hand block. Figures 30–33 shows a push block with your left hand palm down, stepping forward into a right forward stance, giving a spear-hand thrust to the solar plexus and shouting kiai. Before moving, turn your head to the right (see Figure 33 again). You then move your left foot counterclockwise to your left 270 degrees into a left cat stance and left double knife-hand block (see Figures 34–36). Figures 37–38 show stepping with your right foot 45 degrees into a right cat stance and right double knife-hand block. Figures 39–41 show stepping 135 degrees clockwise to your right, ending in a right cat stance with a right double knife-hand block. Figure 42–43 show stepping with your left foot 45 degrees to your left into a left cat stance and left double-hand block.

Figures 44–46 show stepping with your left foot 45 degrees counterclockwise into a left forward stance. From this position, perform a heel palm strike with your right hand while using your left hand, palm outward, to protect your exposed right armpit. Figures 47–54 show performing a forward scooping block with your right hand. Your left hand returns to your left side. Your right hand should finish in a middle block position. Bring your right foot up to your left foot and perform a front snap kick with your right foot at a 45-degree angle to your right. Rechamber and step into a right forward stance (see Figure 54), and then perform a reverse punch with your left hand (do not step forward with your left foot). Figures 55–58 show a fast side-scooping block with your left hand; your right hand is on your right hip. Bring your left foot to your right, maintaining a middle block position with your left hand. Perform a snap kick with your left foot 45 degrees to your left. Rechamber, step into a left forward stance (see Figure 59), and reverse punch (do not step forward with your right foot) with your right hand (see Figure 60). Step directly forward into a right forward stance and execute a right augmented forearm block (see Figures 61–63). Shout "kiai." Turn your head to the right (see Figure 63). Figures 64–69 show moving your left foot counterclockwise 270 degrees ending in a left forward stance while simultaneously performing a down block, and then a high block. (We were taught to perform the next move by opening and closing our left hand while maintaining the high block; however, we have seen the move performed numerous ways.) Step 45 degrees to the right into a right forward stance while simultaneously performing a right high block with your fist (see Figures 70–73). Figures 74–78 show looking over your right shoulder, stepping with your right foot 135 degrees clockwise into a right forward stance while simultaneously executing a right down block, and then performing a right high block. Open and close the right hand. Figures 79–80 show stepping forward with your left foot 45 degrees to your left into a left forward stance while simultaneously executing a left high block with your left forearm. Figures 81–82 show the beginning of the final bow.

This kata, regardless what name different people call it, it is primarily a basic kata with basic movements and should always end *exactly* where it started.

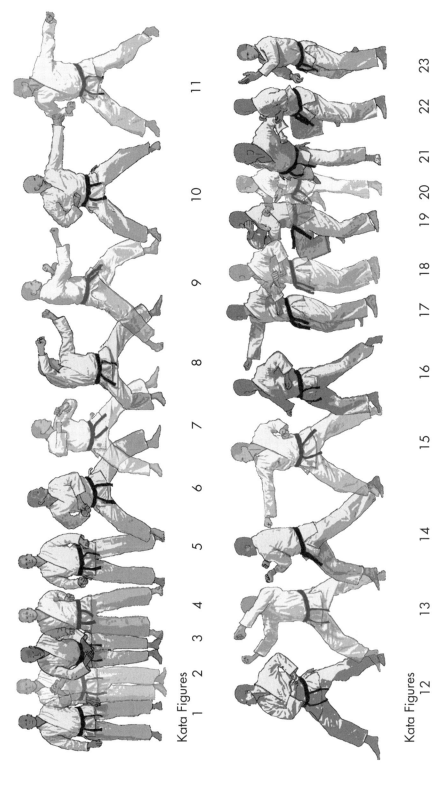

Kata Figures
1 2 3 4 5 6 7 8 9 10 11

Kata Figures
12 13 14 15 16 17 18 19 20 21 22 23

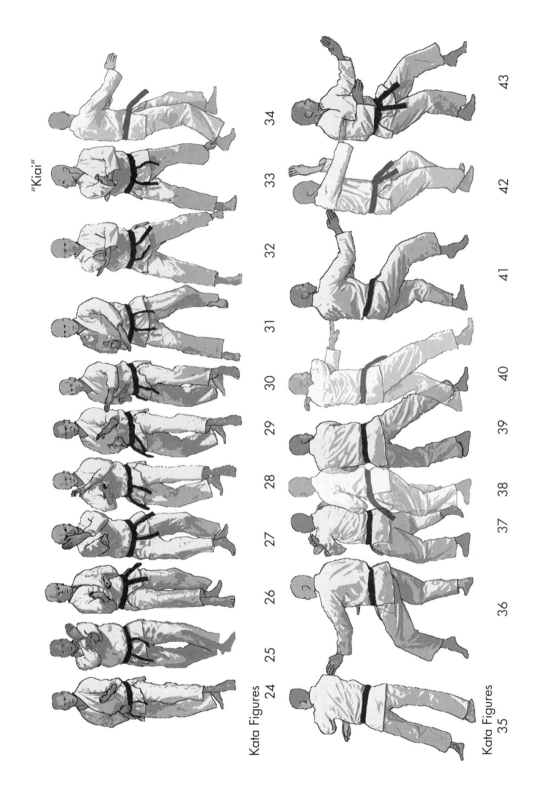

"Kiai"

Kata Figures
24 25 26 27 28 29 30 31 32 33 34

Kata Figures
35 36 37 38 39 40 41 42 43

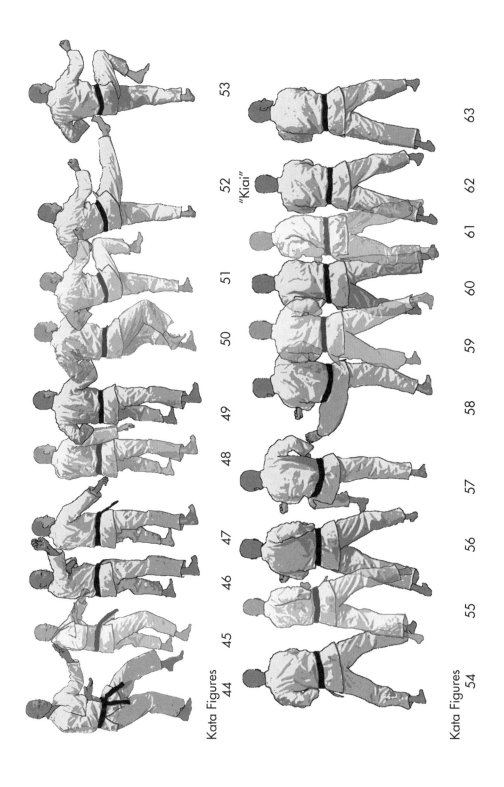

53
52
"Kiai"
51
50
49
48
47
46
45
Kata Figures
44

63
62
61
60
59
58
57
56
55
54
Kata Figures

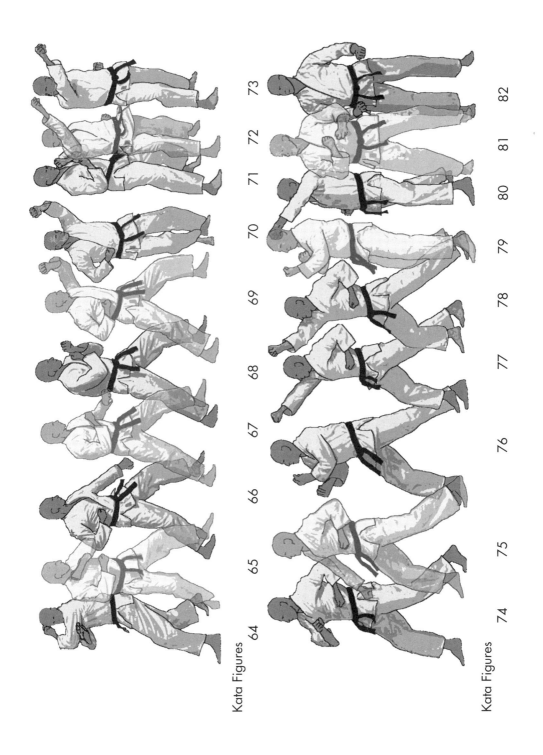

Kata Figures

Kata Figures

64 65 66 67 68 69 70 71 72 73

74 75 76 77 78 79 80 81 82

CHAPTER SEVEN

My Introduction to Kata

My mother and father were the owners of a circus. From my very early childhood, I worked in their circus. And when I say "worked," I mean worked—no playing involved. From the time I was barely old enough to stand, I had a serious role. As a tiny tot I was performing stands on my parent's hands and later I was a tender of the large elephant, Modock, as well as doing whatever other jobs my father instructed me to do.

By age 16, I had had enough of the circus life and ran away to join the United States Marine Corps. I completed boot camp at the tender age of 17 and arrived in Japan on April Fools Day, 1955. My first post was at a converted naval base about eight miles from Yukosaka, Japan.

My introduction to the martial arts occurred four months later. It was rather inauspicious, to say the least. I went into the shower and noticed that I had forgotten my soap. There was another person in the shower and I asked him for his soap. Being a cocky 17-year old fresh out of boot camp, the manner of my request was not overly tactful. The next thing I knew, he had kicked me in the chest, knocking me off of my feet and causing me to slide across the shower floor on my buns until I hit the wall. When I looked up, he was standing over me preparing to strike again. I was cocky but not suicidal, I quickly raised my hand and said "I apologize, keep your soap." He turned and continued his showering. As I rose, my curiosity outweighed my pride, I asked him how he had accomplished such a feat and he replied, "karate." "What the hell is karate?" I asked. He explained that karate was the Japanese method of fighting with empty hands and feet.

You have to remember that this was the mid 1950s. World War II had only been over for a decade and General MacArthur's ban on the practice of the martial arts had only been lifted a few years earlier. Also, before the war, the practice of karate was virtually unknown in the Western world, although many Westerners were familiar with judo and its predecessor, jujitsu. I addressed this gap in my earlier book *Japan's Ultimate Martial Art, Jujitsu Before 1882, The Classical Japanese Art of Self-Defense* (Charles E.

Tuttle Co. Inc., 1995). There were few Westerners who could even spell karate, much less do it. However, the practical demonstration that I had just witnessed intrigued me sufficiently to ask my newfound friend to take me to where he practiced this unusual way of fighting. We got dressed and took one of the rickshaws that waited outside the base into town.

These rickshaws were the old half-motor-powered, half human-powered contraptions. Riding in one was an adventure in itself because the road into town was quite hilly. Consequently, we had to push the thing up the hills and hold on for dear life on the down slopes.

The road into town led first to Souvenir Alley, which is what we called the shop-lined street that catered to the military personnel. At the end of the street was where the red-light district began. At the end of the red-light district, the road turned uphill again. About halfway up this hill, a small wooden frame building sat on blocks. This building, I would come to call a "dojo," and in it I began my formal martial arts training.

I would like to be able to say—as so many other martial artists have written about their beginnings—that from the outset I was a natural; that I trained strenuously and religiously, never being late for or missing a class; that I learned all my katas quickly and proficiently; that I entered and won many tournaments. The truth, I'm sad to say, is different.

At that time, the monthly contribution to the dojo was 120 yen. Since the exchange rate at that time was 360 yen to the American dollar, this meant that my monthly cost for attending was roughly 33 cents. The teacher was Omik Kobayashi, a student of Master Gogen Yamaguchi of the Goju Ryu style. There were never more than eight people training at the dojo at any one time. My shower buddy and I were the only non-Orientals. Lessons were taught in Japanese or Okinawan; since we did not speak either language, they could have been taught in Russian for all we knew. Actually, there was very little spoken instruction, mainly just a lot of point-ing and sign language. They tolerated, but I do not believe they really liked, us being there. I do not remember anyone wearing a uniform at practice. Everyone had a white belt except the teacher and his two assis-tants. I studied there for two and a half years, but I cannot say that I got into karate seriously until later, after my tour in Japan was completed.

Shortly after that my Marine Corps unit was transferred to the Philippines and then on to Okinawa. It was in Okinawa that I began to study karate seriously under Sensei Z. Shimabuku. He was of the Shorin Ryu school. It was also at this time that I was introduced to the Okinawan weaponry that is unique to that string of islands. Shimabuku Sensei was not a big man, but he was very skillful. He taught martial arts in the traditional manner. Today it would be called "old fashioned." That is, he taught what had been handed down through the generations, not something that he had contrived himself, or had been cobbled together from various styles. He taught largely through kata, which we did repeatedly. I'm sure he thought we would never do it correctly. One day Sensei told the class that he was going to teach kai-sei of the kata. I came to know kai-sei as the self-defense application of the kata. Later in my martial arts career, I came to realize that kai-sei was the oyo of karate kata.

I completed my tour of duty and returned to the United States in 1959. I continued my training, first in Houston under the late Sensei M. Richardson of the Seibukan Shorin Ryu, and then under Senseis G. Tong and Lim-Kwa Chwee in California. Senseis Tong and Chwee were students of Sensei Masutatsu Oyama of Japan Kyohushin Kai and it was under them that, in 1965, I was awarded my first black belt.

From time to time, students ask me: "Where did you get all of your training?" I generally respond by saying that I have been fortunate to have trained under some of the finest karate practitioners in the world, but I never took the time to go back and reconstruct when and with whom this training was conducted.

For those students who have inquired, here is the best I can recollect. The senseis I have named below are only those with whom I have had extensive training; that is, long daily sessions over many consecutive weeks or, in several cases, months. I have not attempted to name those who came to my dojo for a few days only, or those I visited for a like amount of time. Because the time span involved is almost 40 years, I am afraid I may have overlooked a few wonderful teachers. To them, I express my profound apologies.

By 1967, I opened, with a friend, my first school, which we called The House of the White Moon. We maintained the House of the White Moon until I opened my current school, The Houston Budokan. In 1968 I began training under Sensei G. Norris, a Shorin Ryu student of Sensei Z. Shimabuku of Okinawa. In 1971, I studied under Sensei R. Baillargeon, who was the United States representative for Seishin Kai Karate Union headed by Sensei Siyogo Kuniba of Osaka, Japan. Sensei Baillargeon was a practitioner of the Shito Ryu style, which I teach today. By 1974, I had become the Texas representative of the Seishin Kai Karate Union.

In 1975, I had the pleasure of having Sensei S. Matsoo, the All Japan Karate Champion, stay at my house and train in my dojo for six months. Sensei Matsoo was a student of Sensei S. Kuniba and Sensei H. Yamada, both of the Motobu-Ha Shito Ryu. Senseis Kuniba and Yamada were both students of Master Kenwa Mabuni, a founder of Shito Ryu, Sensei Syoshin-Nagamine, the founder of Shorin Ryu and Ryusho-Tomoyori, the founder of Kenyu-Ryu. Sensei Kuniba's father, Sensei Kosei Kuniba, was the founder of Seishin Kai and a student of Master Choki Motobu, the founder of Motobu-Ha.

In 1976, I returned to Japan again and studied under Sensei Tsuyos Tagawa of the Shito Ryu school. Two years later I went back to Japan to study further under Sensei Kuniba and Sensei Y. Yamonoka, also of the Shito Ryu style. Two years later I was back again, this time to Kejik University to study under Sensei Hironori Yamada, of the Shito Ryu style, and Sensei S. Yamanaka, of the Iioju Ryu style.

Over the next several years, I was fortunate to have three fine Japanese senseis come to America and train at my dojo. First, there was Sensei Tadahiko Ohtsuka of the Goju Kensha who came in 1983. The following year, Sensei Sokon Ikeda, also of the Gojo Ryu came. In 1986, Sensei Junhi Fukuzawa, a Shito Ryu master, lived and trained at my school for eleven months. 1987 saw me returning to Japan to continue my advancement, this time under the tutelage of Sensei Junichi Iosu, a Shito Ryu master.

As readers of one of my earlier books, *The Heart of Kendo* (Shambala Press, 1999), know, by the late 1960s, I had begun to devote my life fully to the martial arts. During this time, my lifelong passion for kendo, jodo, iaido, taiho-jitsu, judo, aikido and kubodo began to flourish. During the ensuing years, I also studied extensively with masters of these arts as well. Because all of the arts have certain common fundamentals, or because one grew from the other, in most cases these wonderful teachers were masters of several arts. For example, many of the kendo masters were also experts in iai and jodo. Similarly, many of the judo masters were highly proficient in jujitsu and aikido. It would greatly lengthen this chapter, and serve no useful purpose, to attempt to name all of these senseis.

However, to them I am profoundly grateful.

Glossary

Age-zuki: Rising punch.

Ashi: Leg or foot.

Ashi-guruma: Knife-foot kick.

Bara-te: Reverse punch.

Bonno: Loss of focus, also suki or disturbed feeling.

Budo: Growth in spirit through the martial arts.

Budoka: Practitioner of the martial ways, also budo.

Budo-seishin: Martial spirit.

Bunkai: To disassemble and break down to fundamental parts of the application.

Dachi: Stance.

Dan: Grade.

Dojo: Practice hall.

Embusen: Performance line or kata.

Empi: Elbow strike.

Fumi-dashi: Long step.

Funikoshi, Gichin Sensei: Founder of Heian katas.

Gayku-zuki: Reverse punch.

Gi karate: Uniform.

Hachiji-dachi: Open leg stance.

Hajime: Begin, start.

Haragei: Ability to locate and use one's life force.

Heian kata: means peaceful, also same as pinan.

Heijo-shin: Relaxed, calm but focused state of mental awareness.

Heisoku-dachi: Closed-feet stance or attention stance.

Heiwa-antei: Peace and calmness.

Hidari: Left.

Itosu, Anko Sensei: Founder of pinan katas.

Itosu, Yasutsune Sensei: Responsible for the pinan katas being taught to the public rather than behind closed doors.

Jodan: Area of the face or upper body.

Jodan-junzuki: Stepping punch to the face.

Ka: Student practitioner.

Kamae: Posture.

Karate: Form of martial arts from Asia, Japan and Okinawa.

Karateka: A person who practices karate.

Kata: Prearranged and choreographed formal movements or exercises; also means example, moving meditation.

Katate-ushi: Hammer-fist strike also Kentsui-kuchi.

Keage: Snap kick.

Kekomi: Front kick.

Ken: Fist.

Kensei: Silent kiai.

Keri: Kicking.

Ki: An individual's life force.

Kiai: Loud shout originating from the lower abdomen or lower stomach area; yell of spirit.

Kiba-dachi: Horse stance.

Kihon: Basic movements that can be practiced perfectly without conscious thought or effort.

Kime: Ability to focus single-mindedly on the immediate task at hand.

Kohai: A junior, less experienced student.

Kokutsu-dachi: Back stance.

Koshi: Hips.

Kumite: Sparring.

Kuniba, Kosei Sensei: Founder of Seishin-kai style.

Kurai: Flexible and passive state of mind.

Kyu: Lower-class rank, below black belt.

Mae: Front.

Mae-te: Palm strike.

Martial: Derived from Mars, the Roman god of war.

Migi: Right.

Mokuso: Brief period of meditation before starting a kata or class.

Morote-te: Both hands.

Morote-uke: Double forearm block.

Mune: Chest.

Mushin: "No self, no mind", a state of mental clarity.

Musubi-dachi: Informal attention or ready stance.

Nukite: Spear-hand strike.

Oi-zuki: Lunge punch.

Osae-uke: Pressing block.

Otoshi-uke: Blocking with a push.

Rei: Ceremonial bow.

Riken: Back-fist strike.

Seiken: Fist.

Sensei: Teacher.

Shihan: A master or venerable teacher.

Shimei: Strike to a vital point that can dangerous or fatal.

Shizen-tai: Natural posture.

Shuto: Knife hand, when palm is up the inside edge of the hand.

Shuto-uke: Knife-hand block.

Shygyo: Austere training or self analysis.

Suigetsu: Solar plexus.

Sukui-uke: Forearm block.

Tamashiwari: To test one's spirit.

Tan-dien: A point 3 inches below the navel, considered to be the source of a life force, also hara.

Te: Empty as in kara-te, empty hand.

Tsuki: Punch.

Uchi: Striking.

Ue-zoe: To place on top of.

Uke: Blocking or person who attacks.

Uraken: Backfist strike.

Ushiro: Back of or block to the rear.

Waza: Technique.

Yoko: Side.

Yoko-keage: Side snap kick.

Zanshin: To maintain awareness after completion of a technique or kata. To have a perfect finish to one's last movement.

Zanzen: Meditation, reflection.

Zenkutsu-dachi: Forward stance.

Zuki: Punch.

Index

ateru, 29

attackers, 32, 95

Baillargeon, R., 161

Ballerinas and kata, 37-38

black belt, 10-11, 32-33

block, 31-32, 40, 64, 70, 72, 74

body and kata training, 38

bunkai, 2, 7
   applications, 92-94
   as soul of karate, 28
   defined, 6
   demonstrating, 64-66
   first element in kata, 51-52
   in kata, 1, 43, 44-45
   inherent, 32
   Okinawan karate, 28
   oyo and, 52-54, 74, 76

bushi, 9, 26

Chiba Sensei, 42

Chwee, Lim-Kwa, 161

combat, 92-94

contraction of body, 37

defenders, 95

defensive techniques, 40

dojos, 28

ego, 4

empty-hand systems, 26

expansion of body, 37

family fighting systems, 9

fighting systems 9, 26, 26-27, 36

Fukien Shaolin Temple, 8, 26

Fukizawa, Junhi, 162

Fukuda, K., 5, 6, 47, 55

Funikoshi, Gichin, 8, 28, 40

Goju Kensha Ryu, 162

Goju Ryu style, 160

hard control of power, 37

henka, 44, 45
   demonstrating, 78
   third element in kata, 55

hidden moves, 2

hidden techniques, *See also* kakushi

House of the White Moon, 161

Houston Budokan, 161

Iioju Ryu, 162

Ikeda, Sokon, 162

Iosu, Junichi

issen-issatsu, 9, 26

Japan Kyohushin Kai, 161

ju no kata, 47

judo kata in, 47-48

judo, testing standards, 11

jujitsu, 8

kai-sei, 161

kakushi, 44-45
   demonstrating, 80-91
   fourth element in kata, 55-56

Kana, Dr. Jigaro, 10-11

Kano, Dr. Jiro

karate
   as exhibition, 29
   as sports, 29
   development of, 36
   history of, 8
   introduction to Japan, 2
   oral traditions, 27-29
   pronunciation of, 8

karateka, training of, 28-29

kata, 7, 49-50
   Americanization of, 38-39
   as combat with self, 10
   as martial arts, 35
   ballerinas and, 37-38
   bunkai, 1, 3, 5, 41, 43, 45
   bunkai and oyo, 52-54
   changes in, 7, 42
   defensive technique, 40
   elements of, 51-57
   henka, 45
   in judo, 47-48
   kakushi, 44, 45
   language of, 44
   oyo, 47
   practice of, 30-32
   primacy of, 28
   source of, 25, 25-26
   teaching of, 12-13
   training, 4, 9, 38

keiko, 9, 27

kendo, testing standards, 11

Kenyu Ryu, 162

Kobayashi, Omik, 160

Kokuba, Kosei, 28

Konishi, Yasuhiro, 28

kumite, Okinawan karate, 28

Kuniba, Kosei, 162

Kuniba, Siyogo, 161-162

Mabuni, Kenwa, 28, 162

martial arts, 32-33
    ego and, 4
    kata in, 35
mastery, 29, 56
Matsoo, S, 161
mental awareness, 48
mind, 4, 38
Miyagi, Chojun, 28
Motobu, Choki, 8, 162
Motobu-Ha, 162
mushin, 4, 29
Nagamine, Syoshin, 162
Norris, G., 161
novice teachers, 38-39
Ohtsuka, Hironishi, 28
Ohtsuka, Tadahiko, 162
Okinawa, 8, 8-9, 26
Okinawa Te, 8
Okinawan karate, 8, 27-29
Oyama, Masutatsu, 161
oyo, 44, 45, 92-93
    bunkai and, 52-54
    demonstrating, 68-77
    kai-sei, 161
    second element in kata, 53-54
power, 37, 38
punch, 31-32
ranking systems, 10, 10-11
Richardson, M., 161
Ryobu-Kan dojo, 28
samurai, 8, 9, 26
satori, 4
secret teachings 26-28, *See also* kakushi
Seibukan Shorin Ryu, 161
Seishin Kai, 162
self-defense, 32, 92
self-improvement, 32
Shimabuku, Z., 160
Shito Ryu, 161, 162
Shorin Ryu school, 160, 162
soft control of power, 37
sparring, 4, 5, 6, 36
speed, 37, 37-38
sports, 29-30
students, 12-13
styles of karate, 3
swords, 93-94
Tagawa, Tsuyos, 162
teachers, 12, 12-13, 36-39

Tomoyori, Ryusho, 162
Tong, G., 161
tools as weapons, 26
tournaments, 30, 30-31, 57
traditional kata, 2
training, kata, 28-29, 31-32
uchikomi, 6
visualization, 32
waza, 9, 27, 95-157
weapons, 26
Yamada, H, 161-162
Yamada, Hironori, 162
Yamaguchi, Gogen, 160
Yamanaka, S., 162
Yamonoka, Y., 162
zanshin, 48

BOOKS & VIDEOS FROM YMAA

YMAA Publication Center Books

B041/868 101 Reflections on Tai Chi Chuan
B031/582 108 Insights into Tai Chi Chuan—A String of Pearls
B046/906 6 Healing Movements—Qigong for Health, Strength, & Longevity
B045/833 A Woman's Qigong Guide—Empowerment through Movement, Diet, and Herbs
B009/041 Analysis of Shaolin Chin Na—Instructor's Manual for all Martial Styles
B004R/671 Ancient Chinese Weapons—A Martial Artist's Guide
B015R/426 Arthritis—The Chinese Way of Healing and Prevention (formerly Qigong for Arthritis)
B030/515 Back Pain—Chinese Qigong for Healing and Prevention
B020/300 Baguazhang—Emei Baguazhang
B043/922 Cardio Kickboxing Elite—For Sport, for Fitness, for Self-Defense
B028/493 Chinese Fast Wrestling for Fighting—The Art of San Shou Kuai Jiao
B016/254 Chinese Qigong Massage—General Massage
B057/043 Chinese Tui Na Massage—The Essential Guide to Treating Injuries, Improving Health, & Balancing Qi
B038/809 Complete CardioKickboxing—A Safe & Effective Approach to High Performance Living
B021/36x Comprehensive Applications of Shaolin Chin Na—The Practical Defense of Chinese Seizing Arts for All Styles
B010R/523 Eight Simple Qigong Exercises for Health—The Eight Pieces of Brocade
B025/353 The Essence of Shaolin White Crane—Martial Power and Qigong
B014R/639 The Essence of Taiji Qigong—The Internal Foundation of Taijiquan (formerly Tai Chi Chi Kung)
B017R/345 How to Defend Yourself—Effective & Practical Martial Arts Strategies
B013/084 Hsing Yi Chuan—Theory and Applications
B056/108 Inside Tai Chi—Hints, Tips, Training, & Process for Students & Teachers
B033/655 The Martial Arts Athlete—Mental and Physical Conditioning for Peak Performance
B042/876 Mind/Body Fitness
B006R/85x Northern Shaolin Sword—Forms, Techniques, and Applications
B044/914 Okinawa's Complete Karate System—Isshin-Ryu
B037/760 Power Body—Injury Prevention, Rehabilitation, and Sports Performance Enhancement
B050/99x Principles of Traditional Chinese Medicine—The Essential Guide to Understanding the Human Body
B012R/841 Qigong—The Secret of Youth
B005R/574 Qigong for Health and Martial Arts—Exercises and Meditation (formerly Chi Kung—Health & Martial Arts)
B040/701 Qigong for Treating Common Ailments—The Essential Guide to Self-Healing
B011R/507 The Root of Chinese Qigong—Secrets for Health, Longevity, & Enlightenment
B055/884 Shihan-Te—The Bunkai of Kata
B049/930 Taekwondo—Ancient Wisdom for the Modern Warrior
B032/647 The Tai Chi Book—Refining and Enjoying a Lifetime of Practice
B019R/337 Tai Chi Chuan—24 & 48 Postures with Martial Applications (formerly Simplified Tai Chi Chuan)
B008R/442 Tai Chi Chuan Martial Applications—Advanced Yang Style (formerly Advanced Yang Style Tai Chi Chuan, v.2)
B035/71x Tai Chi Secrets of the Ancient Masters—Selected Readings with Commentary
B047/981 Tai Chi Secrets of the Wǔ & Li Styles—Chinese Classics, Translations, Commentary
B054/175 Tai Chi Secrets of the Wu Styles—Chinese Classics, Translations, Commentary
B048/094 Tai Chi Secrets of the Yang Style—Chinese Classics, Translations, Commentary
B007R/434 Tai Chi Theory & Martial Power—Advanced Yang Style Tai Chi Chuan (formerly Advanced Yang Style Tai Chi Chuan, v.1)
B022/378 Taiji Chin Na—The Seizing Art of Taijiquan
B036/744 Taiji Sword, Classical Yang Style—The Complete Form, Qigong, and Applications
B034/68x Taijiquan, Classical Yang Style—The Complete Form and Qigong
B046/892 Traditional Chinese Health Secrets—The Essential Guide to Harmonious Living
B039/787 Wild Goose Qigong—Natural Movement for Healthy Living
B027/361 Wisdom's Way—101 Tales of Chinese Wit

YMAA Publication Center Videotapes

T004/211 Analysis of Shaolin Chin Na
T007/246 Arthritis—The Chinese Way of Healing and Prevention
T028/566 Back Pain—Chinese Qigong for Healing & Prevention
T033/086 Chin Na In Depth—Course One
T034/019 Chin Na In Depth—Course Two
T008/327 Chinese Qigong Massage—Self Massage
T009/335 Chinese Qigong Massage—With a Partner
T012/386 Comprehensive Applications of Shaolin Chin Na 1
T013/394 Comprehensive Applications of Shaolin Chin Na 2
T005/22x Eight Simple Qigong Exercises for Health—The Eight Pieces of Brocade
T017/280 Emei Baguazhang 1—Basic Training, Qigong, Eight Palms, & Their Applications
T018/299 Emei Baguazhang 2—Swimming Body & Its Applications
T019/302 Emei Baguazhang 3—Bagua Deer Hook Sword & Its Applications
T006/238 The Essence of Taiji Qigong—The Internal Foundation of Taijiquan
T010/343 How to Defend Yourself 1—Unarmed Attack
T011/351 How to Defend Yourself 2—Knife Attack
T035/051 Northern Shaolin Sword—San Cai Jian and Its Applications
T036/06x Northern Shaolin Sword—Kun Wu Jian and Its Applications
T037/078 Northern Shaolin Sword—Qi Men Jian and Its Applications
T029/590 The Scientific Foundation of Chinese Qigong—A Lecture by Dr. Yang, Jwing-Ming
T003/203 Shaolin Long Fist Kung Fu—Gung Li Chuan and Its Applications
T002/19x Shaolin Long Fist Kung Fu—Lien Bu Chuan and Its Applications
T015/264 Shaolin Long Fist Kung Fu—Shi Zi Tang and Its Applications
T025/604 Shaolin Long Fist Kung Fu—Xiao Hu Yuan (Roaring Tiger Fist) and Its Applications
T014/256 Shaolin Long Fist Kung Fu—Yi Lu Mai Fu & ɪr Lu Mai Fu and Their Applications
T021/329 Simplified Tai Chi Chuan—Simplified 24 Postures & Standard 48 Postures
T022/469 Sun Style Taijiquan—With Applications
T024/485 Tai Chi Chuan & Applications—Simplified 24 Postures with Applications & Standard 48 Postures
T016/408 Taiji Chin Na
T031/817 Taiji Sword, Classical Yang Style—The Complete Form, Qigong, and Applications
T030/752 Taijiquan, Classical Yang Style—The Complete Form and Qigong
T026/612 White Crane Hard Qigong—The Essence of Shaolin White Crane
T027/620 White Crane Soft Qigong—The Essence of Shaolin White Crane
T032/949 Wild Goose Qigong—Natural Movement for Healthy Living
T023/477 Wu Style Taijiquan—With Applications
T020/310 Xingyiquan—The Twelve Animal Patterns & Their Applications
T001/181 Yang Style Tai Chi Chuan—and Its Applications

YMAA PUBLICATION CENTER 楊氏東方文化出版中心

4354 Washington Street Roslindale, MA 02131
1-800-669-8892 • ymaa@aol.com • www.ymaa.com